PROJECTION, IDENTIFICATION, PROJECTIVE IDENTIFICATION

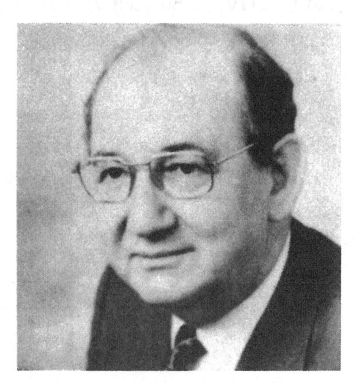

Joseph Sandler

PROJECTION, IDENTIFICATION, PROJECTIVE IDENTIFICATION

Edited by

JOSEPH SANDLER

Freud Memorial Professor of Psychoanalysis
in the University of London

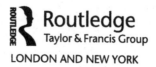

Routledge
Taylor & Francis Group

LONDON AND NEW YORK

First published 1988 by Karnac Books Ltd.

Published 2018 by Routledge
2 Park Square, Milton Park, Abingdon, Oxon OX14 4RN
711 Third Avenue, New York, NY 10017, USA

Routledge is an imprint of the Taylor & Francis Group, an informa business

British Library Cataloguing in Publication Data
A C.I.P. for this book is available from the British Library

ISBN: 9780946439409 (pbk)

To my children, Trudy, Catherine, and Paul — those
excellent vehicles for projection, identification and
projective identification.

Contents

Contributors

Yoram Bilu, Ph.D., Senior Lecturer, Department of Psychology, The Hebrew University of Jerusalem.

Betty Joseph, Training and Supervising Analyst, British Psycho-Analytical Society.

Otto F. Kernberg, M.D., Associate Chairman and Medical Director, The New York Hospital - Cornell Medical Center, Westchester Division; Professor of Psychiatry, Cornell University Medical College; Training and Supervising Analyst, Columbia University Center for Psychoanalytic Training and Research.

W. W. Meissner, S. J., M.D., Clinical Professor of Psychiatry, Harvard University; Training and Supervising Analyst, Boston Psychoanalytic Institute.

Rafael Moses, M.D., Training and Supervising Analyst, Israel Psychoanalytic Society, Jerusalem.

Meir Perlow, M.A., Research Fellow, Sigmund Freud Center of the Hebrew University of Jerusalem.

Joseph Sandler, Ph.D., M.D., LL.D., Freud Memorial Professor of Psychoanalysis in the University of London; Training and Supervising Analyst, British Psycho-Analytical Society.

Contents

Foreword

The papers and discussions in this book are the fruits of the First Conference of the Sigmund Freud Center of the Hebrew University of Jerusalem. The conference was held at the Hebrew University during my tenure as Sigmund Freud Professor of Psychoanalysis, and papers were presented by W. W. Meissner, Betty Joseph, Otto F. Kernberg, and Rafael Moses. These are all to be found in this volume. But in addition to the program as originally arranged, a paper of special interest, on dybbuk possession, was given by Dr. Yoram Bilu, a distinguished anthropological psychologist. Further material has also been included. An introductory chapter presenting an overview of the concepts of internalization and externalization, by Meir Perlow and myself, represents an expanded version of material circulated but not read at the conference. The book continues with a specially added chapter on projective identification, in which the development of the concept is traced through three major stages, presenting it in terms comprehensible to those lacking a Kleinian psychoanalytic background.

I was privileged to take the chair throughout the conference, and was thus able to ensure a continuity in the discussions which might not have been possible had we followed the more usual procedure of having a different chairperson for each session. My special thanks are due to the staff of the Sigmund Freud Center for the tremendous amount of work they put into the organization of this most successful conference. I want to acknowledge in particular the skill and dedication of the indefatigable Administrative Director of the Center, Hannah Groumi, who organized and supervised every detail of the meetings. Special thanks are owed to Michele Morowitz, who undertook the difficult and tedious task of transcribing the recordings of the conference discussions. The editing of the final manuscript was done in London, and I want to express my gratitude to Jane Pettit for reading through the material, making numerous corrections, and assembling and checking the references. My thanks are due also to Bryony Tanner, who did the final typing and checking.

The conference and this book would not have seen the light of day were it not for the work done by the contributors, who performed a most difficult task in quite exemplary fashion.

Joseph Sandler
University College, London
June 1986

Chapter 1

Internalization and Externalization

JOSEPH SANDLER AND MEIR PERLOW

In the early years of psychoanalysis, particularly because of the influence of Karl Abraham, there was a tendency to consider processes of internalization and externalization in concrete terms such as "taking in" or "putting into the other person." This tendency has continued in certain groups of psychoanalysts, especially those influenced by the work of Melanie Klein and Wilfred Bion. While many may disagree with such concrete formulations of psychological processes, it should be borne in mind that such reification may be extremely useful from the point of view of description. We are throughout dealing with *concepts*, with theoretical constructs whose value should be considered primarily in terms of their clinical utility.

A specific direction of development pertinent to the ideas we are considering is that taken by ego psychology, greatly influenced by the postwar work of Heinz Hartmann, Ernst Kris, Rudolph Loewenstein, Edith Jacobson, and others. On the basis of their work a major distinction is now regularly made between the ego as a "structure" or "apparatus," on the one hand, and the "self-representation," i.e., the mental representation of oneself, on the other. In this context "self" is analogous to "object," and "self-representation" parallels the mental representation of the object (Sandler and Rosenblatt, 1962; Sandler, 1986).

The psychoanalytic terms that can be grouped under the broad headings of externalization and internalization overlap considerably, and it is our purpose here to comment briefly on such terms as projection, identification, introjection, and incorporation, in preparation for the papers and discussions to follow. Because of the current interest in

1

projective identification, Chapter 2 has been devoted entirely to a discussion of that concept.

PROJECTION

This term was used in various ways by Freud and subsequent writers. In its most general sense it could be said to have been regarded by Freud as the tendency to search for an outside cause rather than an internal one, and this is reflected as early as 1895 in Draft H (Freud, 1887–1902), where, writing of paranoia in a female patient, Freud remarks that the purpose of the illness is "to fend off an idea that was intolerable to her ego by projecting its subject-matter into the external world" (p. 111). In this context Freud refers to projection as a "transposition" and comments that in the illness there is an "abuse of a psychical mechanism which is very commonly employed in normal life." He goes on to say, "Whenever an internal change occurs, we can choose whether we shall attribute it to an internal or external cause. If something deters us from accepting an internal origin, we naturally seize upon an external one" (p. 111). Freud speaks here of the "misuse of the mechanism of projection for purposes of defence" (p. 112), but he tended later to consider projection a mechanism of defense in its own right, i.e., as the defensive attribution of unwanted thoughts, wishes, feelings, and related mental contents to some other person. Naturally Freud's references to projection as a defense were especially related to paranoia (1896, 1911, 1915a, 1922) and jealousy (1922).

Projection was seen by Freud as central also to the construction of phobias (see, e.g., Freud, 1915b, 1916–1917, 1917, 1926). In the phobia the instinctual threat, endangering the ego from within, is "projected" into external reality, where it can more readily be controlled by phobic avoidance. Thus he states (1915c):

> by means of the whole defensive mechanism . . . a projection outward of the instinctual danger has been achieved. The ego behaves as if the danger of a development of anxiety threatened it not from the direction of an instinctual impulse but from the direction of a perception, and it is thus enabled to react against this external danger with the attempts at flight represented by phobic avoidances. [p. 184]

In addition to the usages mentioned above, Freud also employed the term in the more general sense of directing or turning "outward." So we find, for instance, in "The economic problem of masochism" (1924) the statement that "We shall not be surprised to hear that in certain circumstances the sadism, or instinct of destruction, . . . has been directed outwards, projected, . . ." (p. 164).

Freud (1917) spoke of the dream as "a *projection*: an externalization of an internal process" (p. 223), and in *Totem and Taboo* (1912–1913) referred to projection as

> a primitive mechanism, to which . . . our sense perceptions are subject, and which therefore normally plays a very large part in determining the form taken by our external world. . . . internal perceptions of emotional and thought processes can be projected outwards in the same way as sense perceptions; they are thus employed for building up the external world, . . . owing to the projection outwards of internal perceptions, primitive men arrived at a picture of the external world which we, with our intensified conscious perception, have now to translate back into psychology. [p. 64]

At this point it is perhaps sufficient to mention that Freud used the term projection in a variety of other contexts as well, including religion (1912–1913, 1927) and even space (1941). A full account of Freud's use of the term in his prepsychoanalytic writings has been given by Ornston (1978). It is worth noting that in 1909 Ferenczi proposed that projection (he referred to it as "primal" projection) was involved in what we would now call the infant's differentiation of self from the external world, and this use of the term was taken over by Freud.

It is possible to follow the development of the projection concept after Freud in two main directions. The first reflects the emphasis placed by psychoanalysts on projection as a mechanism of defense (A. Freud, 1936), and the term has a variety of meanings within that context (see Hendrick, 1936; Knight, 1940; Waelder, 1951; Novick and Kelly, 1970). The differences in the various definitions of projection as a defense have led to the extraction of a notion of "projection proper," seen as "a defense against a specific drive derivative directed toward an object" and "motivated by the sequence of fantasied dangers consequent upon drive expression" (Novick and Kelly, 1970, p. 84).[1] However, the elasticity of the projection concept is such that it would, in our view, be unwise to tie a definition of projection "proper" to defense against a drive derivative, and

---

[1] For a discussion of the concept in relation to "projective testing" see Bellak (1950).

it seems more appropriate to regard it as a relatively wide concept, the meaning of which is dependent on the context in which the term is used. The elasticity of the concept is not, however, confined to projection, and it will be seen that very similar problems of definition arise in relation to the other concepts subsumed under the general headings of internalization and externalization.

From a representational standpoint the distinction between "inner" and "outer" is one which has been built up within the representational world of the child (Sandler and Rosenblatt, 1962), and in consequence all the varieties of projection have to be seen as involving a displacement of mental content from a self-representation to an external object representation, to a representation of an aspect of the world that is "not-me." In its simplest form it would be the attribution of an unwanted aspect of one's self-representation to a mental representation of another person, i.e., to an object representation. This does not involve the condition that projection need be specifically related to an unwanted *impulse* or that it be regarded as "reflexive," i.e., that the impulse be directed back toward the subject from whom it originates.

The second major direction of development in regard to projection is that taken by Melanie Klein and her followers. Following from Ferenczi's original thoughts about projection as a process of assigning unpleasant aspects of experience to the outer world (1909), she strongly emphasized the view of projection as the process whereby the ego expelled (projected) its own sadistic impulses into the external world (Klein, 1930, 1931). Klein's conception of mental processes as being intimately related to fantasies (a view stated systematically by Susan Isaacs, 1948, and expounded clearly by Hanna Segal in 1973) contributed to her view of the close relation between projection and anal fantasies of expulsion. So the concept of projection came to be closely related to—indeed, it could almost be said to be equated with—the fantasy of the expulsion of (poisonous) feces into the mother or her breast.

A number of major differences in contemporary views on the concept of projection remain to be mentioned. One of these has been touched on earlier, i.e., differences in regard to the "reflexive" quality to be attributed to the mechanism. Another major area of disagreement centers around the question of whether a self-object boundary is necessary for projection to take place.[2] Proponents of the view that there is no such boundary at the beginning of life consider projection (in its defensive

[2]For an extensive discussion of the contemporary clinical usage of the concept see J. Sandler's discussions on the topic with Anna Freud (Sandler, 1985).

aspects, at least) to be incapable of occurring very early: as there is no boundary for the unwanted content to "cross over," this content cannot be allocated to the "nonself." This issue is linked to the degree and "depth" of the pathology thought to be associated with the use of projection. Finally, we should mention the problem of the influence of projection on the object onto (or into) which it has occurred. This problem is closely related to the question of projective identification, discussed extensively in Chapter 2. In practice, projection is not always fully differentiated from projective identification.

EXTERNALIZATION

This term has been widely used as a synonym for projection in its various senses. Freud certainly used it in this way when referring to projection in its most general meaning, that of putting some unwanted content outside oneself. This has been referred to earlier in relation to the dream (1917, p. 223). However, in recent years the term has been used rather more specifically, and a number of writers have discussed a distinction between the terms projection and externalization.

One of the more specific uses of the latter term relates to Anna Freud's notion of "externalization of conflict" (A. Freud, 1936, 1965). This refers to the transformation of an internal conflict (especially so-called intersystemic conflict, i.e., conflict between the inner agencies of id, ego, and superego) into conflict with an external object. Externalization of this sort has been regarded both as a normal, everyday phenomenon and as an element of the transference situation in analysis. An example of everyday externalization of conflict would be the externalization of the superego onto some individual who would become a figure of authority with whom the person might be in conflict (this has, of course, also been called "projection of the superego"). Similarly, and somewhat more patho-logically, someone may externalize his id and feel that people around him are trying to seduce him. We must confess that the difference between externalization of this sort and some form of projection is hard to see, although the emphasis on the "putting outside" of internal *conflict* may be the important element in the distinction.

More recently research has been devoted to the relation between externalization and transference phenomena (A. Freud, 1965; Sandler, Kennedy, and Tyson, 1975, 1980; Furman, 1980). Anna Freud (1965) clearly distinguishes externalizations from object relationships (and there-fore from transference) in the analysis of children:

> Not all the relations established or transferred by a child in analysis
> are object relations in the sense that the analyst becomes cathected
> with libido or aggression. Many are due to externalizations, i.e., to
> processes in which the person of the analyst is used to represent one
> or the other part of the patient's personality structure. [p. 41]

However, she goes on to say, in relation to adult analysis, that

> The analyst of adults is not unfamiliar with the externalization of
> intersystemic as well as intrasystemic conflicts in his patients. Severe
> obsessional neurotics stage quarrels between themselves and their
> analyst about minor matters to escape from painful inward indeci-
> sions caused by ambivalence. Conflicts between active and passive,
> masculine and feminine strivings are externalized by attributing the
> wish for one of the two possible solutions to the analyst and fighting
> him as its representative. [p. 42]

Anna Freud then lists further clinical varieties of externalization and
adds, "Understood in this manner, externalization is a subspecies of
transference. Treated as such in interpretation and kept separate from
transference proper, it is a valuable source of insight into the psychic
structure" (p. 43). Many analysts nowadays would find it extremely
difficult to trace the dividing line between externalization in analysis and
"transference proper," a distinction made more difficult by the increasing
realization that transference (and object relations) cannot simply be
equated with the cathexis of the analyst with libido or aggression, but
involves multiple elements, including many which are noninstinctual.

One use of "externalization" deserves special mention. This is the
"putting out" of the so-called internal objects or introjects which form a
fundamental part of the internal world. With the concept of "dialogue
with the introject" (Sandler and Sandler, 1978), the externalization of an
aspect of the introject onto (or into) the analyst as part of transference (as
opposed to the externalization or projection of an aspect of the self-
representation) has received increased attention. This phenomenon is,
however, not a new one (see Fairbairn, 1941; Bychowski, 1956) and has
been referred to by Eduardo Weiss as "extrojection" (1947). The sharp
distinction between the externalization or projection of an aspect of the
self-representation and the externalization of an object representation has
not been made in any systematic way by Kleinian authors, although it is
reflected in the work of such writers as Racker (1968), who examined
different forms of countertransference.

In an attempt to differentiate externalization from projection, it has been suggested that use of the former term be restricted to the involvement of the non-drive and object-bound aspects of the self-representation (Novick and Kelly, 1970). The developmental implications of this formulation have also been explored (Furman, 1980). Other suggestions made in regard to the definition of externalization have included one by Brodey (1965), who has extended the definition to include the manipulation of the external object in order to make it comply with what the subject is attempting to externalize. This would bring the concept within the boundaries of contemporary uses of the notion of projective identification. The suggestion has also been made that the term be used as a "blanket" term to cover all forms of attributing some aspect of one's internal world or one's psychic structure to the outside.

INTERNALIZATION

With this term we enter into the realm of the various concepts used to describe processes of "taking in." "Internalization" is often used as a blanket or umbrella term in this context, to embrace such concepts as introjection, incorporation, and identification. The overlapping and changing meaning of the latter terms has been repeatedly discussed in the literature, and the concept of internalization has itself been the object of critical discussion (Strachey, 1941; Schafer, 1972; Grossman, 1982). In light of this, it seems that the most convenient use for the term is the blanket one, to cover all forms of "taking in," and it is in this sense that we shall use it.

Freud did not distinguish strictly between the various forms of internalization. On the whole he used the term in connection with two related processes. The first of these was the internalization of external prohibitions and regulations (Freud, 1927, 1930, 1931, 1933a, 1939). The second was in reference to the internalization of aggression, the turning of aggressive impulses inward, i.e., back toward the self (1930, 1933a, 1933b, 1933c). Both sets of processes were considered to be intimately involved in the establishment of the superego. There are a few other infrequent uses of the term by Freud. Examples may be found of its use in relation to the perception of a danger as being located internally (1926), and to the "taking in" of an external stimulus (1915a).

In 1939, in *Ego Psychology and the Problem of Adaptation*, Heinz Hartmann extended Freud's conceptualizations of internalization to take into account a developmental process whereby the individual becomes increasingly independent of his environment. In the process of internalization the person adopts as his own certain behavior which previously appeared only as a direct reaction to environmental stimulation. Hartmann considered the development of thinking, of the superego, and of methods of mastering internal danger to be examples of this process. The broadness of the concept, and the confusion in the literature about the meaning of "internal" led to a number of attempts to differentiate aspects of the concept of internalization. Thus a distinction has been made between internalization in the sense used by Hartmann and the "organizing activity" involved in the developing perceptual and cognitive activities of the child (Sandler, 1960). Hans Loewald (1962) has distinguished between processes leading to the establishment of the boundary between self and object (primary internalization) and subsequent processes of "taking in" (secondary internalization). Loewald (1962, 1980) has also stressed the point that it is *relationships* that are internalized, relationships which exist first with external objects and then, after internalization, become intrapsychic. In 1967 David Rapaport was led by Hartmann's broad conceptualization of internalization to propose a distinction between the "inner" world of mental representations and the "internal" world of psychic structure. He proposed limiting the term internalization to those processes which affect the inner world, differentiating internalization from incorporation, introjection, and identification, processes involving the internal world.

Anna Freud makes use of the concept primarily in relation to the "taking in" of external conflict (1965) and in this context distinguishes internal conflict (conflict between opposing instinctual wishes) from internalized conflict. In *Aspects of Internalization* Schafer (1968) emphasizes internalization as the taking over of the motives of the object. All these views reinforce the suggestion that internalization be used as a general term for all forms of "taking in."

IDENTIFICATION

Freud made use of the term identification in some of his earliest letters to Fliess (1887–1902) and shortly afterward in *The Interpretation of Dreams* (1900). Freud clearly used the term in two quite different senses. He spoke of hysterical identification, in which the symptom is formed on the basis of identification with some aspect of another person, but spoke also of identification in dreams, a phenomenon in which two persons, linked by some element shared in common, appear as a single figure in the manifest content.

With the development of Freud's interest in narcissism (1914), an interest which led eventually to the formulation of the structural theory (1923), the concept of identification gained in importance. No longer simply a process whereby symptoms or dream elements were formed, identification came to be recognized as an important developmental process. As such, it was considered by Freud to be related to the oral instinctual impulse of *incorporation* (following a suggestion made by Abraham), and to the mental counterpart of this oral impulse, i.e., *introjection* (after Ferenczi). Both these terms came to be closely related to the notion of identification in Freud's writings, at times being used synonymously.

Freud distinguished a number of different types of identification (e.g., hysterical and narcissistic) linked particularly with melancholia and superego formation. He saw it both as a developmental step connected with the resolution of the oedipus complex and as a central process in character formation. Freud's use of the concept is complicated by the fact that its meaning varied according to context, that it was not properly differentiated from other forms of internalization, and that he did not differentiate identification leading to ego (and "self") development from identifications contributing to superego formation.

Much has been written on identification since Freud, and it has been seen both as a normal developmental mechanism and as a mechanism of defense. Views range from those emphasizing very early, oral instinctual trends to those stressing processes that assume the existence of an established self-representation. It would be an impossible task to review the literature on identification here, but it seems worthwhile to propose a distinction between primary and secondary identification based on formulations involving self- and object representations (Sandler and Rosenblatt, 1962).

Primary identification.   In representational terms this could be said to relate to the state which exists before a firm boundary between self and object (or self- and object representations) has been established. It has also been described (Sandler, 1960) as a state of primary identity or primary confusion, in which the infant cannot differentiate the representational aspects of his own self from those of the object. In relation to pathology, the state of primary identification has been described as a regressive one in which "de-differentiation" of self and object occurs and so-called "ego boundaries" ("self boundaries") have been lost or put out of action. This is most commonly seen in severe psychotic states (Jacobson, 1964). However, a "fleeting primary identification" or "fleeting confusion" between self and object has been described as a ubiquitous normal phenomenon

(Sandler, 1961; Sandler and Joffe, 1967). This phenomenon relates to what Weiss has called "resonance identification" (1960), which can be regarded as a basis of empathy.

Secondary identification. This is probably the most common meaning of the term identification. During this process the representational boundary between self and object is not lost, but the subject embodies in the self-representation attributes of the object, real or fantasied. In this sense of the term it can be regarded as the vehicle for so-called secondary narcissism, in which admiration, love, and esteem for the object are transferred to one's own self (a process which in the past was often referred to by such phrases as "incorporating the object into the ego"). In Kleinian usage this is "introjective identification."

Many types of identification have been described, the most prominent of which is Anna Freud's concept of identification with the aggressor (1936). Others include counteridentification (Fliess, 1953), pseudoidentification (Eidelberg, 1938), concordant and complementary identifications (Racker, 1957), and adhesive identification (Bick, 1968).

Introjection. It should be said at the outset that this term is often used to refer to all forms of internalization, including identification. It was introduced originally by Ferenczi (1909, 1912), who used it to refer to all the processes whereby the ego forms a relationship with an object, thereby including that object within the ego. This encompassed *"every sort of object love* (or *transference*) both in normal and in neurotic people" (Ferenczi, 1912, p. 316). While Freud eventually adopted the term, he generally used it for the process of setting up the parents, in the mind of the child, as the superego (1924), or for the internalization of the lost object in melancholia. (Freud also referred to these processes as identification!) Following Abraham (1924), emphasis was placed by many psychoanalytic writers on the instinctual aspect of introjection, and it was frequently referred to as the psychic process analogous to the infant's oral incorporation at the breast (Fenichel, 1925, 1926; Fuchs, 1937). However, the defensive aspect of introjection has also been stressed in the literature (Rapaport, 1967).

It seems to us useful to distinguish between (1) the use of "introjection" to refer to the perceptual "taking in" of the external world; (2) the use of the term to refer to the construction of an important object in the child's fantasy world (the "introject") which provides him with, for example, feelings of the reassuring "presence" of the object (see Weiss, 1939; Sandler, 1960; Schafer, 1968); and (3) superego introjection, occurring later, in which the parental objects (modified by projections and other fantasy distortions) are "set up" in the mind of the child as his superego (Sandler, 1960).

From a representational point of view it is valuable to make a sharp distinction between identification as a modification of the self-representation on the one hand, and introjection as the setting up of unconscious, internal "phantom" companions, felt to be part of one's inner world, yet external to one's self-representation, on the other. If this distinction is accepted it would be legitimate to speak of "identification with the introject," through which one feels identified with some aspect of one's superego introjects and is enabled to take up a moral stance toward others. (It should be noted that the terms introject and internal object are often used synonymously.)

INCORPORATION

In addition to its use as a synonym for other forms of internalization, "incorporation" was used rather more specifically by Freud (1933a) to refer to the aim of the oral instinct. He had considered it the "prototype" of later processes of identification (1905), but the emphasis on the oral aspect of internalization was reinforced by Abraham, who took the view that all forms of internalization could be regarded as derived from oral incorporative impulses (1924). Later attempts to gain more precision in regard to the term centered around the question of whether it should be restricted to the biological act of taking something in through an orifice, usually the mouth. Proponents of this view included Fenichel (1925, 1926), Greenson (1954), and Sandler and Dare (1970). Others have considered it appropriate for the term to include reference to the incorporation wish or fantasy (Schafer, 1968; Meissner, 1981). Kleinian usage has consistently been both to use incorporation in the sense of oral taking in, and to equate this with all forms of internalization. It is still a matter of controversy whether *all* identifications can be considered to be derived from fantasies of incorporation.

A number of authors have emphasized the close relation between incorporation and fantasies of merging (e.g., Fenichel, 1926; Searles, 1951; Guntrip, 1952; Jacobson, 1964) and fantasies of destroying the object (Freud, 1918; Klein, 1975b). From a representational point of view it would seem that a clear distinction can be made between the *physical act* of incorporating and *fantasies or thoughts* of incorporation, conceived of by the individual as an act of physical "taking in."

Chapter 2

The Concept of Projective Identification

JOSEPH SANDLER

The introduction of the concept of projective identification by Melanie Klein in 1946 was set against a rather confused and confusing background of literature on various forms of internalization and external-ization—imitation, identification, fantasies of incorporation, and many varieties of projection. Projective identification is a broad concept, as the following description by Hanna Segal (1973) indicates:

> In projective identification parts of the self and internal objects are split off and projected into the external object, which then becomes possessed by, controlled and identified with the projected parts.
>
> Projective identification has manifold aims: it may be directed towards the ideal object to avoid separation, or it may be directed towards the bad object to gain control of the source of danger. Various parts of the self may be projected, with various aims: bad parts of the self may be projected in order to get rid of them as well as to attack and destroy the object, good parts may be projected to avoid separation or to keep them safe from bad things inside or to improve the external object through a kind of primitive projective reparation. Projective identification starts when the paranoid-schizoid position is first established in relation to the breast, but it persists and very often becomes intensified when the mother is perceived as a whole object and the whole of her body is entered by projective identification. [pp. 27–28]

In this context Segal explicitly treats projective identification as a mech-

13

anism of defense, but elsewhere she describes it as "the earliest form of empathy" and as providing "the basis for the earliest form of symbol-formation" (p. 36). Melanie Klein saw it as the vehicle for distinguishing "me" from "not-me" (Klein, 1946). Rosenfeld (1965) has described processes entering into psychotic states and comments that "Melanie Klein described these primitive object relations and the ego disturbances related to them under the collective name 'projective identification'" (p. 158). Over the past thirty-five years, projective identification has become increasingly seen by Kleinian analysts as a central mechanism in counter-transference, and in this context Bion's addition of the container-contained model has played a specially important part (Grinberg, Sor, and de Bianchedi, 1977). Ogden (1979, 1982) has emphasized the role of projective identification as the pathway from the intrapsychic to the interpersonal.

It is possible to cite many other ways in which the concept of projective identification has been employed, and it is clear that its "collective" and necessarily "elastic" nature must render any precise definition implausible. But it must be equally clear that the term has carried with it an idea which has proved to be of substantial value to a significant group of analysts. It has become a central Kleinian clinical concept, though it is also used by analysts with other orientations. However, it is a notion that is difficult to discuss from a non-Kleinian perspective. This may in part be due to the fact that those who use the concept tend to speak of it as a single mechanism, while in fact it is one which (like so many others in psychoanalysis) shifts its meaning according to context. It has as a result acquired a certain mystique, with the unfortunate consequence that it is sometimes either dismissed entirely or thought to be understandable only with special "inside knowledge."

This paper refers to my own attempts to come to grips with the concept, and I have no doubt that I will be seen by some to have done violence to it. Because my own frame of reference differs in significant respects from that of the Kleinians, it has been necessary to break the concept down in my own mind in order to digest and absorb it. For the sake of convenience I shall present the material that follows under a number of different headings. Like all concepts in psychoanalysis, that of projective identification has undergone a progressive development since its introduction. It is convenient to separate this development into three stages. These are, I believe, conceptually clear-cut, although they overlap considerably, and the ideas of the first and second stages have persisted alongside those of the third.

THE BACKGROUND

In the period between the two world wars, and particularly after the mid-twenties, processes of internalization and externalization became increasingly important in psychoanalytic thinking. These processes were particularly evident in psychotic patients, and this led Melanie Klein to construct and elaborate a theory of development in which object relationships were seen as being built up on the basis of these internalizing and externalizing processes. She distinguished the two "positions" in normal development on the basis of the two major psychotic states in which these processes could be seen most clearly. Although one might disagree with Mrs. Klein's theory of development and with the concrete nature of her formulations, in retrospect we can see that she was the analyst who gave the earliest and greatest recognition to projective and identificatory processes in the development of object relationships, and to their operation in the here-and-now of the transference. I believe that it was *clinical* pressure which prompted this development, and in this context it is interesting to note that Anna Freud has remarked, in her work on the mechanisms of defense (1936), that she was prompted to develop her ideas by the need to understand resistances in analysis more fully. In relation to Anna Freud's introduction of a number of new defenses in 1936, I have commented elsewhere (Sandler, 1983) that

> what Anna Freud did at this time was to introduce a whole class of what might be called object-related defences, which involved reversal of roles or some combination of identification and projection. These are defences in which there is an active interchange between aspects of the self and of the object, the unacceptable aspects of one's own self being dealt with by producing (or attempting to produce) their appearance in the external object. Often, simultaneously, frightening or admired aspects of the object may be taken into the self. [p. 41]

FIRST STAGE PROJECTIVE IDENTIFICATION

When Melanie Klein introduced the term projective identification in 1946, she wrote:

> Much of the hatred against parts of the self is now directed towards the mother. This leads to a particular form of identification which establishes the prototype of an aggressive object-relation. I suggest for

these processes the term "projective identification." When projection is mainly derived from the infant's impulse to harm or to control the mother, he feels her to be a persecutor. In psychotic disorders this identification of an object with the hated parts of the self contributes to the intensity of the hatred directed against other people. [p. 102]

Although this formulation was put by Mrs. Klein in very concrete terms, it can be understood as referring to processes which occur *in fantasy*, processes of change in the mental representation of self and object occurring at various levels of unconscious fantasy. The concreteness of the formulations can be taken to refer to processes *imagined* as concrete, i.e., involving images of literal incorporation or of "forcing" something into an object. The processes described are defensive or adaptive in the immediate present, although when they occur in extreme form in infancy they may have harmful effects on later development. Melanie Klein can be taken to be referring here to shifts and displacements within the child's representational world (Sandler and Rosenblatt, 1962). *Identification* with parts of an object can be regarded as a "taking into" the self-representation aspects of an object representation. Projection is then a displacement in the opposite direction, i.e., aspects of the self-representation are shifted to (and made part of) an object representation. In my view it does not matter very much, in this context, whether we speak, for example, of "the bad parts of the self" or of "the hated (or despised) unwanted aspects of the self-representation," as long as we agree that the processes described by Mrs. Klein occur within fantasy life. Moreover, in my view, for conceptual purposes we can separate the idea of projective identification as a *mechanism* operating in the here-and-now from processes described in the Kleinian theory of early development. I shall touch on this point again later, but I want to emphasize that what is of the greatest importance for me in Mrs. Klein's formulation is her description of a mental mechanism or set of mechanisms. For Melanie Klein projective identification involved splitting, which I would understand in this context as a splitting-off of parts of the self-representation or of the object representation. Projective identification involves projection in that it is an identifying of the object with split-off parts of the self. When the process moves in the opposite direction, i.e., toward identifying oneself with aspects of the object, Mrs. Klein speaks of introjective identification.

I speak here of *first stage projective identification* in order to emphasize the point that for Mrs. Klein projective identification was a process that occurs *in fantasy*. Let me put it another way. The real object employed in the process of projective identification is not regarded as being affected—the parts of the self put into the object are put into the fantasy object, the "internal" object, not the external object. This is borne out by the way in which transference and countertransference are treated in Mrs. Klein's writings. Transference reflects infantile object relationships (Klein, 1952) and is *a fantasy about the analyst* which needs to be analyzed. It is a fantasy that creates a distortion of the patient's perception of the analyst, a distortion based on, among other things, the projective identification that has affected the patient's fantasy about the analyst. Countertransference, in its turn, is scarcely mentioned, and when it is—e.g., in *Envy and Gratitude* (1957)—it is regarded as a hindrance to the analyst's technique.

SECOND STAGE PROJECTIVE IDENTIFICATION

It was probably inevitable that the concept of projective identification came to be widened soon after its introduction, and I want to touch here on a particular extension of the concept to object relationships in general and to the transference-countertransference relation between patient and analyst in particular. In 1950, Paula Heimann (then very much a Kleinian) drew attention to the positive value of countertransference thoughts and feelings in analysis. "The analyst's countertransference is an instrument of research into the patient's unconscious" (p. 84), she wrote. "From the point of view I am stressing, the analyst's counter-transference is not only part and parcel of the analytic relationship, but it is the patient's *creation*, it is part of the patient's personality" (p. 83).

It is of interest that a number of writers made a very similar point at about this time, some linking countertransference specifically with projective identification. Thus Racker, in a series of papers beginning in 1948 (Racker, 1968), connected the analyst's countertransference response to projective identification on the part of the patient. In regard to a case he was discussing, he said:

> the "projective identification" . . . frequently really obtains its ends—in our case to make the analyst feel guilty and not only implies (as has been said at times) that "the patient expects the analyst to feel guilty," or that "the analyst is meant to be sad and depressed." The analyst's identification with the object with which the patient identifies him, is, I repeat, the normal countertransference process. [p. 66]

Racker makes a valuable distinction in this context between *concordant* and *complementary* identification on the part of the analyst. To put it simply, countertransference based on a concordant identification occurs when the analyst identifies with the patient's own fantasy self-representation of the moment. Countertransference based on a complementary identification occurs when the analyst identifies with the object representation in the patient's transference fantasy.

Heimann, Racker, and others such as Grinberg (1957, 1958, 1962) made a significant extension of projective identification by bringing it into conjunction with the analyst's identification with the self- or object representation in the patient's unconscious fantasies, and with the effect of this on the countertransference. The countertransference reaction could then be a possible source of information for the analyst about what was occurring in the patient.

I have called the formulations referred to above *second stage projective identification* because they represent an extension of Melanie Klein's original propositions, whereas projective identification occurring within the person's fantasy life (reflected in a fantasy distortion of the analyst), can be called first stage projective identification. If either the self or the object represented in such unconscious fantasies is identified with by the analyst to a degree sufficient to contribute to the analyst's countertransference, we have an instance of second stage projective identification.

THIRD STAGE PROJECTIVE IDENTIFICATION

In this stage of the development of the concept it is no longer one or the other aspect of the unconscious fantasies that is identified with by the analyst. Projective identification is now described as if the externalization of parts of the self or of the internal object occurs directly *into* the external object. This extension was given its main impetus by the work of Bion in the late fifties and found explicit expression in his concept of the "container" (1962, 1963). Bion describes the function of the container by presenting what is essentially Melanie Klein's description of projective identification, to which he adds the following (Grinberg, Sor, and de Bianchedi, 1977):

> One of the consequences of this process is that, by projecting the bad parts (including fantasies and bad feelings) into a good breast (an understanding object), the infant will be able—insofar as his development allows—to reintroject the same parts in a more tolerable form, *once they have been modified by the thought (reverie) of the object* . . . . [p. 29; italics mine]

By no stretch of the imagination can this be understood as occurring in fantasy only, nor is this what Bion intended to imply. What he describes here is a concrete "putting into the object." He says:

> An evacuation of the bad breast takes place through a realistic projective identification. The mother, with her capacity for reverie, transforms the unpleasant sensations linked to the "bad breast" and provides relief for the infant who then reintrojects the mitigated and modified emotional experience, i.e., reintrojects . . . a non-sensual aspect of the mother's love. [p. 57]

Bion's formulations can be related to Winnicott's "holding" function of the "good enough mother" (1958), and are echoed too in aspects of Ogden's conception (1982). What Bion has proposed in the container-contained metaphor is clearly of great relevance for analytic technique, and I shall return to this projective identification later.

It must be clear that all the theoretical propositions put forward in connection with transference and countertransference apply equally to object relationships outside the analytic situation.

COMMENTS

The comments that follow relate to various aspects of projective identification, and are somewhat disjointed. However, they will give an indication of my own view of projective identification.

1. An integral part of Kleinian theory is that which relates to very early infantile development, and to early object-relations. Later adult functioning is seen as rooted in this particular developmental view. In consequence, Kleinian formulations regarding adult mental processes tend to be couched in concepts used to describe infantile ones. However, I believe it mistaken to assume that the idea of projective identification *as a mechanism* is part of a package which includes a theory of development and which has to be accepted in its entirety. Nor need we be put off by the concreteness of metaphors used, for we all use metaphors in our theory (and in our interpretations), and what is important is to be aware that we *are* using metaphors. Consequently I have no difficulty in absorbing Mrs. Klein's description of projective identification (first stage projective identification) into my own frame of reference, in which it can be regarded as a mechanism involving shifts and displacements in mental representation or in fantasy. I would put emphasis on its role as a *mechanism* for regulating unconscious feeling states and emphasize, too, that

this mechanism can be divorced if necessary from the specific fantasy content associated with projective identification by Mrs. Klein and her followers. Let me stress, however, that together with the Kleinians, I believe that processes of projective identification (in the sense in which I can make use of them) play a highly significant part in development and in the clinical psychoanalytic situation. Projective identification has given an added dimension to what we understand by transference, in that transference need not now be regarded simply as a repetition of the past. It can also be a reflection of fantasies about the relation to the analyst created in the present by projective identification and allied mechanisms.

2. The element of *control* of the objects (into which parts of the self have been projected) has been consistently stressed by Kleinian writers on projective identification, and it is an element which is, I believe, central to the concept. What one wants to get rid of in oneself can be disposed of by projective identification, and through controlling the object one can then gain the unconscious illusion that one is controlling the unwanted and projected aspect of the self. The urge to control the object is evident in the process of "living through another person"—Anna Freud's "altruistic surrender" (1936) can be taken as a good example of this process. But there is a further aspect of the wish to control the object which is worth stressing. It is a common clinical observation that patients who feel guilty ("attacked by an internal persecutor") may deal with the guilt and gain powerful narcissistic supplies by projecting the guilty ("bad") part of the self onto another, while at the same time identifying (by "introjective identification") with the persecutor. This provides a double gain, i.e., the gain of identifying with the (usually idealized) part of the superego introject as well as that of getting rid of the "bad" unwanted part of the self. This gives a powerful motive for control of the object into which the projective identification has taken place (Sandler, 1960).

3. I have made use of the phrase "into the object" rather than "onto." For many years, of course, projection "into" was Kleinian usage, and non-Kleinians took care to speak of "projection onto." However, if we accept that projection is a process that involves self- and object *representations*, then we need have no difficulty in accepting the phrase "into the object." But this does not mean, in my view, that we have necessarily to accept the idea that projective identification is accompanied by fantasies of entering and invading. However, the idea of "forcing" an aspect of oneself into the object raises no difficulty because projective identification as a mechanism of defense aims at reducing anxiety, and this is a strong motive for applying force to keep the projected aspect on the other side of

the self-object boundary. This force is reflected in the resistance shown by patients to accepting projected aspects of the self back into the self-representation.

4. The role of the self-object boundary is clearly important in projective identification and deserves a few comments. For projective identification to function as a mechanism of defense the existence of a boundary between self and object is essential so that a person can feel dissociated from the split-off parts of the self. Because in psychotic states it is difficult to maintain representational boundaries, projective identification may be intensified as an attempt to establish them. If they cannot be established, a state of panic may follow. It is worth noting that although we, *as observers*, may see the massive use made of projective identification in certain psychotic states, for the psychotic the existence of a persecutor in his fantasies means that he has (perhaps only temporarily) established a self-boundary of sorts. Here I find myself in disagreement with those who tend to see projective identification as a psychotic mechanism only. While in psychosis it may be massive, it is nevertheless ubiquitous; it might also be preferable, in line with this, to speak of *pathogenic* rather than pathological projective identification.

5. It has been stated (Klein, 1946) that projective identification is a mechanism whereby the boundary between self and object is established in infancy. This notion of projective identification is difficult to reconcile with the requirement of a self-object boundary for successful projective identification. I would suggest that the concept need not be applied to these early differentiating processes, but, if it is, it could be understood as referring to the differentiation of mental representations of self and object in a way which is different from projective identification as a mechanism of defense. What I mean is that we can conceive of *attempts* at projection and identification (or, perhaps better, identification and disidentification) occurring as the infant struggles to organize what has been regarded as a state of primary confusion between experiences of self and object, and thereby to gain control over his feeling states. These attempts can be taken to contribute, in their turn, to the gradual establishment of self and object boundaries.

6. If we turn now to *second stage projective identification* we must immediately be concerned with the relation between a *fantasy* of the object (the object representation) as modified by projective identification and its effect on a real external person. This is, as has been pointed out by many, most evident in the dimension transference-countertransference.

Within my own frame of reference it is insufficient to say that the internal fantasy object is "put into" the analyst. Rather, I understand the process as follows:

a. A fantasy is created, involving the analyst. Projective identification enters into the creation of the fantasy, which is a *wishful* one, i.e., it has behind it a pressure toward gratification or fulfillment.

b. The patient attempts to actualize (Sandler, 1976b) the unconscious wishful transference fantasies, to make them real, to experience them (either overtly or in disguised form) as part of reality. He will do this in numerous ways in the analytic situation, some of which will evoke a countertransference response which can be meaningful to the analyst in the ways described by Heimann, Racker, Grinberg and others. In a previous paper (Sandler, 1976a) relating to actualization and object relationships, I commented on the wishful fantasy as follows:

> it involves a self-representation and object-representation, and an interaction between the two. There is a role for both self and object. Thus the child who has a wish to cling has, as part of this wish, a mental representation of clinging to someone else; but he also has, in his wish, a representation of the object responding to his clinging in a particular way. Those role relationships which appear in the transference are representative of the important wishful aspect of the unconscious fantasy life. This is rather different from the idea of a wish consisting of a wishful aim being directed towards an object. A notion of an aim which seeks gratification needs to be amplified by an idea of a wished-for role interaction, *with the wished-for or imagined response of the object being as much a part of the wishful fantasy as the activity of the subject in that wish or fantasy.* ... it can be said that the patient in analysis attempts to *actualize* the role relationship inherent in his current dominant unconscious wish or fantasy, and that he will try to do this (usually in a disguised and symbolic way) within the framework of the analytic situation. ... it is not a great step to say that the striving towards actualization is part of the wish-fulfilling aspect of all object relationships. I do not use the term *actualization* here in the same sense as it is used by a number of other psychoanalytic authors, but quite simply in the dictionary sense, that is, as a making actual; a realization in action or fact. [pp. 64–65]

This quotation relates to the evocation of a response in the analyst which reflects in some way the role of the object in the current wishful fantasy of the patient. This would correspond to Racker's notion (1968) of the analyst's *complementary identification* with the fantasied object of the active internal object relationship. The *concordant identification*, on the other hand, can be said to be the analyst's identification with the self-representation involved in the patient's wishful fantasy. However, I want to suggest that countertransference response due to second stage projective identification is *always* based on identification with a fantasy object, and that when it appears to be identification with aspects of the self-representation, a further intrapsychic step has occurred in the patient's fantasying process, i.e., *a further projective identification* has taken place into a new fantasy analyst-object which then contains projected aspects of the self.

7. The central contribution to *third stage projective identification* is that of Wilfred Bion, and the container model is of substantial clinical and theoretical interest. What I understand by it, in my own frame of reference, is the capacity of the caretaking mother to be attentive to and tolerant of the needs, distress, and anger as well as the love of the infant, and to convey, increasingly, a reassurance that she can "contain" these feelings and, at an appropriate time, respond in a considered and relevant way. Through this the infant learns that his distress is not disastrous, and by internalizing the "containing" function of the mother (through identification or introjection) gains an internal source of strength and well-being. The "reverie" of the mother is to be distinguished from an immediate "reflex" response to the child. The latter process does not require the identification with the child's distress in the same way as does the "reverie" of the "containing" mother.

As far as the analytic situation is concerned, there is a parallel with the description given for the mother and infant. The analyst as "container" is, as I see it, the analyst who can tolerate the patient's distress, hostility, and love—indeed, all his fantasies and feelings—and who as a consequence of his "reverie" can return them to the patient in the form of interpretations which will allow the patient to accept as aspects of himself those parts he had previously considered dangerous and threatening, and which had been dealt with defensively, with ensuing cost. What I find unacceptable is the notion that this process is one of projective identification, unless the concept is stretched to extreme limits. We would have to say, for example, that the child's cry of distress is "put into" the mother by projective identification, and it seems to me that this represents a caricature of the original concept. The "container" model can, I believe, be fruitfully separated from the developmental theory to which it is attached,

as well as from the concept of projective identification (although what the
analyst will "contain" will encompass the patient's transference projections as well as his distress), and has value in its own right. In this regard the
following comments (Sandler and Sandler, 1984) are relevant:

> to achieve what we regard as the aim of the analytic work we need to
> bring the patient to the point where he can tolerate, in a safer and
> more friendly fashion, the previously unacceptable aspects of himself.
> In order to do this he will need to gain insight, in an emotionally
> convincing manner, not only into the content of his unconscious
> fantasies, but also into the nature of what, for present purposes, we
> shall refer to as his "inner world," i.e., his unconscious relation to his
> introjects, with whom he had a continual unconscious internal
> dialogue . . . , his unconscious anxieties and conflicts as well as his
> methods of resolving such conflicts. This includes, of course, an
> understanding of his own usual defensive mechanisms and manoeu-
> vres, with particular reference to the projections and externaliza-
> tions that occur in his unconscious phantasy life—the spectrum of
> mechanisms that have come to be called projective identification. To
> the extent that we can achieve our analytic aims we will . . . be able to
> bring about the reduction of conflict and associated painful affects,
> and to permit a deflection of what was not previously tolerated near
> consciousness into conscious or preconscious thought and phantasy.
> . . . it is our task to work with the patient in such a way that as much
> as possible of the content of what has come close to the surface layers
> . . . can be made readily available to consciousness. In our work we
> strive to bring about the liberation of such material through appro-
> priate interpretations, particularly the interpretation of conflict. But
> because what we have available is the adult form of the relevant
> unconscious content, in order to anchor the progressive mapping of
> the patient's inner world and the central and recurring themes in his
> present unconscious, we have also to reconstruct the patient's past in
> a relevant way, just as much as we have to make constructions about
> his current inner world (which is, of course, a direct descendant of
> the inner world he formed in childhood); and we link the two
> together. [pp. 375–376]

8. Projective identification has been regarded as the basis for
empathy, but without amplification a simple statement of this sort has
little explanatory power. The state of primary confusion between self and

object referred to earlier (usually called primary identification) is one which persists in modified form throughout life, and which can provide the basis for the capacity for empathy. Some time ago W. G. Joffe and I (Sandler and Joffe, 1967) advanced the following formulation in a paper on the tendency to persistence; I have taken the liberty of quoting from it at length because of its relevance to projective identification:

> Identification (we refer here to secondary identification), as a number of authors now see it, involves a change in the self-representation on the model of an object-representation; and projection is the attribution to an object-representation of some aspect of the self-representation. These processes can occur after the boundaries between self- and object-representations have been created; before that, we have the state referred to by Freud as primary identification, "adualism" by Piaget and primary identity by others. A better term to designate this early state might be "primary confusion". . . . If we apply the idea of persistence to processes of identification and projection in the older child or adult, we can postulate that there will always be a momentary persistence of the primary state of confusion, however fleeting, whenever an object is perceived or its representation recalled. What happens then is that the boundaries between self and object *become imposed* by a definite act of inhibiting and of boundary-setting. It is as if the ego says "This is I and that is he." This is a very different idea from that of a static ego boundary or self-boundary which remains once it has been created. What develops . . . is the ego function of *disidentifying*, a mental act of distinguishing between self and object which has to be repeated over and over again; and the function of disidentifying makes use of structures which we can call boundaries. The persistence of this genetically earlier primary confusion in normal experience is evident when we think of the way in which we move and tense our bodies when we watch ice skaters, or see a Western. We must all surely have had the experience of righting ourselves when we see someone slip or stumble. In these everyday experiences there is a persistence of the primary confusion between self and object; and this may more readily occur in states of relaxation or of intense concentration in which the bringing into play of boundary-setting may temporarily be suspended or delayed. . . . The persistence of this genetically early state . . . must surely provide the basis for feelings of empathy, for aesthetic appreciation, for forms of transference and countertransference in analy-

sis. . . . And in connection with what we call secondary identification and projection, we would suggest that the bridge to these processes is the persisting momentary state of primary confusion or primary identification which occurs before the process of "sorting out" or "disidentifying" occurs. One result of this "sorting out" may be that aspects of the object-representation are incorporated into the self-representation and vice-versa. [pp. 268–269]

The existence of fleeting primary identifications after infancy can give us a tool for improving our understanding of processes of projective identification, for the notion of persistence allows us to account for the fact that we must, in some way, be aware *that what we have projected is our own in order to feel the relief of being rid of it*. I would suggest that in all forms of defensive projection there is a constant to-and-fro, an alternation between the momentary state of "oneness," of primary identification or primary confusion, and the "sorting out" referred to earlier. This would allow one to feel that what is projected is fleetingly "mine," but then, reassuringly, "not mine."

I want to end these comments by expressing some concerns which I am sure are shared by others. First, because projective identification is more a descriptive than an explanatory concept, and because its range of meaning is wide, its use without further elaboration provides a ready pseudoexplanation. Such pseudoexplanations are tempting, and we should be on our guard against them. If projective identification is used as an explanation, its specific meaning in the relevant context should, I think, always be given. Second, because of the close link between the concept of projective identification and our extended understanding of countertransference, it is tempting to see all feelings, fantasies, and reactions of the analyst to his patient as being an outcome of what the patient has "put into" the analyst by means of projective identification. Unfortunately, the differentiation of what belongs to the patient and what to the analyst is likely to remain with us for some time as a difficult technical problem.

Chapter 3

Projection and Projective Identification

W. W. MEISSNER

PROJECTION/INTROJECTION

We can do no better in providing ourselves a starting point and a point of orientation for the ensuing discussion than by returning to the original notion of projection provided by Freud himself. Freud's discussion of the Schreber case (1911) focuses on Schreber's paranoid delusions and the role of projection in his symptom formation. Freud is obviously more secure in his grasp of the formalities and functions of projection than of the nature of the mechanism itself. He regards projection as a mechanism of symptom formation, but his comments lead us only to the threshold of an understanding of projection and little further. He comments as follows:

The most striking characteristic of symptom-formation in paranoia is the process which deserves the name of *projection*. An internal perception is suppressed, and, instead, its content, after undergoing a certain kind of distortion, enters consciousness in the form of an external perception. In delusions of persecution the distortion consists in a transformation of affect; what should have been felt internally as love is perceived externally as hate. We should feel tempted to regard this remarkable process as the most important element in paranoia and as being absolutely pathognomonic for it, if we were not opportunely reminded of two things. In the first place, projection does not play the same part in all forms of paranoia; and, in the second place, it makes its appearance not only in paranoia but under other psychological conditions as well, and in fact it has a regular share assigned to it in our attitude towards the external

27

world. For when we refer the causes of certain sensations to the external world, instead of looking for them (as we do in the case of others) inside ourselves, this normal proceeding, too, deserves to be called projection. [p. 66]

It is generally agreed that projection is the characteristic and basic defense mechanism employed in paranoid states. It is quite obvious clinically that projection is found quite consistently in a variety of other clinical conditions (Jaffe, 1968), so that we cannot regard it simply as a defining or pathognomonic aspect of paranoid states.

Freud put considerable emphasis on projection in trying to illumine the psychodynamics of paranoid delusions. The paranoid deals with painful or intolerable inner impulses by projecting them onto external objects. The process can be rationalized in terms of the economic principle that it is easier to avoid and flee a threatening external source of pain than to avoid an internal one (Nunberg, 1955); but it is not immediately evident why this should be the case.

Looking at projection in its broadest terms, Rapaport (1952) has described it as a structuring of the world in subjective terms according to an organizing principle, inherent in the individual personality, that seeks to diminish internal stress. This encompasses a variety of subtypes: (1) infantile projection by which whatever is painful is externalized; (2) transference processes which may include projective elements; (3) defensive projection of inner impulses, usually paranoid in form; and finally (4) the structuring of the inner world as reflected in projective testing. The subjective structuring has to do with the internalization of introjects which are then projected; they help the infant to structure his world and to define the limits of self and the boundaries between what is within and what is without.

The mechanism of projection can be considered meaningfully only in the context of its correlated intrapsychic process—introjection. The two processes are intimately related in the psychic economy. While psychoanalysts, following Freud, have focused primarily on the role of projection in paranoia, there has been a tendency to overlook or underplay the equally important though less apparent role of introjective mechanisms. The importance of this consideration, both in understanding paranoid mechanisms and in weighing clinical intervention, has been underlined by Searles (1965). On the basis of extensive clinical experience, he comments:

Conspicuous as the defence mechanism of projection is in paranoid schizophrenia, I have come to believe that the complementary defence, introjection, while less easily detectable, is hardly less important. The patient lives chronically under the threat, that is, not only of persecutory figures experienced as part of the *outer* world, but also under that of *introjects* which he carries about, largely unknown to himself, within him. These are distorted representations of people which belong, properly speaking, to the world outside the confines of his ego, but which he experiences—in so far as he becomes aware of their presence—as having invaded his self. These, existing as foreign bodies in his personality, infringe upon and diminish the area of what might be thought of as his own self—an area being kept small, also, by the draining off into the outer world, through projection, of much affect and ideation which belongs to his self. [p. 467]

Projection and introjection are reciprocally related processes which regulate the individual's interaction with external objects. They become operative very early in the organism's experience and remain an operative feature in varying degrees for the rest of life.

It is difficult to indicate starting points for the operation of projection and introjection, but it must be extremely early in life. Klein has specified these processes in the first few months of life (Rosenfeld, 1983). She is undoubtedly correct in pointing to the operation of these mechanisms, but whether they operate in the manner she describes is a matter of controversy. The operation of projective and introjective mechanisms requires a certain degree of differentiation in intrapsychic structure—certainly enough to support a minimal degree of differentiation between self- and object representations. Projection involves an attribution of parts of the self-representation to an object representation; introjection involves a reciprocal attribution of parts of object representations to the self-representation. At the same time, projection and introjection are in part responsible for the emerging differentiation between self and object.

At their most primitive level, these processes are relatively unstructured and undifferentiated. It is impossible to know what the content of such neonatal processes might be or what degree of awareness they might include. Freud's speculation that projection has primarily to do with the operation of the pleasure principle and that the organism responds to maintain an inner pleasurable state—the purified pleasure ego—is probably near the mark. But it is difficult to know whether at this primitive level the processes involved are defensive or not. Klein insists that they are, but they may be serving the interests primarily of differentiation and development, and may only subsequently be put to the uses of defense. At this level, internalizing and externalizing processes may be differentiating rather than defensive processes, and thus directed to the formation and establishment of boundaries between the inner and the outer worlds, between self and object. They would then be the fundamental processes through which internality and externality are constituted. Once these fundamental differentiations are established, the same operations would then be caught up in the commerce between the internal and the external.

The structuring of the inner world begins from the very first. Incorporative aspects of the infant's global and undifferentiated experience precede the capacity to distinguish between self and object, but contribute a qualitative modification to the global experience. The experience is good or bad, or perhaps both, and to the degree that it is unpleasurable leads to primary attempts at externalization, which organize the emerging lines of differentiation. As these lines begin to form, introjection becomes possible and the continuing structuralization of the inner world takes place through introjective mechanisms. The quality of the introjects is derivative from and constituted by elements from both the inner and the outer worlds. What is introjected is qualitatively determined by the characteristics of the real object in conjunction with the elements attributed to it which derive from the inner world. The introject, as I have discussed elsewhere (Meissner, 1970), functions after the manner of a transitional object—it represents a combination of derivatives from the inner and the outer worlds which are assimilated to the inner world.

What is internalized through introjection is a function of an interaction between the real qualities of the object and qualities attributed to it which derive from the subject's inner world. This attribution is projection. The quality of introjects, then, depends in part on the qualities projected from the inner world of drive and instinctual derivatives. To the extent that hostile and destructive instincts are projected on the object, the object becomes a bad, threatening object, so that introjection of that object creates a bad, threatening introject. Similarly, projection of good, loving impulses can help provide good and loving introjects. The quality of the introject, however, is mitigated by the response of the object. A good and loving object can absorb significant amounts of aggressive projective affect and in a sense neutralize it, so that the introject is modified in the direction of ambivalence. Aggressive impulses thus become less threatening, and the infant's capacity to tolerate rage is increased. A hostile, rejecting object, however, can intensify the destructive and threatening quality of the introject, so that the internally destructive aspects of aggression are intensified.

The interplay of introjective and projective mechanisms weaves a pattern of relatedness to the world of objects and provides the fabric out of which the individual fashions his own self-image. Out of this interplay also develops his capacity to relate to and identify with the objects in his environment. It also determines the quality of his object relations. Projection and introjection must be seen in a developmental and differentiating perspective that does not merely reduce them to defense mechanisms. Particularly in the early course of development, they serve important developmental functions. They are intimately involved in the gradual emergence of self and object differentiation and in determining the quality of one's self-image and self-perception, as well as of object relations. Jacobson (1964) has described this aspect of the functioning of these mechanisms:

> During the preoedipal-narcissistic stage, gross primitive introjective and projective mechanisms, in conjunction with pleasure-unpleasure and perceptive experiences, participate in the constitution of self and object images and, hence, of object relations. The small child's limited capacity to distinguish between the external and internal world, which is responsible for the weakness of the boundaries between self and object images and the drastic cathectic shifts between them, promotes the continuous operation of introjective and projective processes. Thus, it is quite true that during the first years of life the child's self and object images still have more or less introjective and projective qualities. [pp. 46–47]

The developmental and defensive aspects of introjection and projection are intertwined. As development progresses, however, differentiation intrapsychically as well as between subject and object reaches a point at which further development depends on the emergence of other, more highly integrated and less drive-dependent processes. The persistence of projection and introjection beyond this point suggests that they are being employed in the service of defensive needs, rather than facilitating the interaction between subject and object. This defensive use serves both to build the structure of the inner world through internalization and to give quality to the experience of the outer world through projection. The persistence of introjective and projective mechanisms in the work of development extends at least through the resolution of the oedipal situation, since introjection and projection are involved in the formation of the superego and the ego ideal. A case can be made that these processes are also significantly involved in the more definitive reworking of the self-organization in adolescence.

The complex interplay of introjection and projection in structuring the inner and outer worlds is modified by the structuring effects of identificatory processes and the resulting emergence of a stable self. As the self becomes organized and stabilized, there is a corresponding definition of the structure, limits, and inherent stability of objects. Perception of the world becomes less drive-dependent, less organized in terms of defensive needs. The capacity for reality testing and tolerance for the distinctness and difference of objects matures.

One way of looking at projection is that it involves a partial differentiation or fusion of self- and object representations (Jacobson, 1964). The infantile interplay between introjection and projection is involved in efforts to define and establish the boundary between self and object, and such fusion and confusion are undoubtedly part of the problem. In later defensive projections, however, such confusions are not apparent and patients seem to be hypersensitive to differences between themselves and others, particularly the objects of their projections. Attribution to the object of characteristics deriving from aspects of the self does not necessarily connote fusion of representations. Rather, in the defensive use of projection the distinction between self and object is amplified in the interest of putting greater distance between the self and what it seeks to reject.

Projection does not involve a withdrawal of cathexis and does not imply a breakdown in cognitive functioning. It implies a careful attention to reality and to the object of projection. The distortion of reality it introduces is not a perceptual distortion. The distortion has rather to do with what the perception means. A significance deriving from inner convictions and needs is attached to what one perceives. Thus, projection does not distort apparent reality but does distort its significance. In short, projection is a form of interpretive distortion of external reality (Shapiro, 1965).

The defensive use of projection can take a variety of forms. An attribute or quality that lies wholly in the subject is perceived as entirely a quality of the object. Conflict is resolved by ascribing to the other person or group the emotions, attitudes, or motives that actually belong to the subject person or group. This use of projection involves a considerable degree of denial and a severe degree of distortion in the perception of external reality. Projection may also take the form of an exaggeration or emphasis of qualities in the other which the subject possesses as well. The degree to which the subject is able to acknowledge the quality in himself varies, but the projection characteristically involves its accentuation in the other. Allport (1958) calls this "mote-beam" projection. Freud (1922) had pointed out that projection of this kind was often involved in jealousy, in which one partner may minimize his own impulses to infidelity while accentuating those of the other. Projection, however, need not take the form of either creating or exaggerating qualities in the other. It may simply take the form of providing an explanation and a justification for an inner state of mind by an appeal to external influences or the imagined intentions and motives of others.

Projection is a defense that pertains primarily to object relations. The content of projection derives from introjects that are in turn derived from object relations. Moreover, projection is immediately caught up in the affectual involvement in object relations. Jaffe (1968) has pointed to the dualistic and conflictual role of projection in involving the self in a persistent mode of ambivalence in dealing with others. At one pole annihilation of the object is sought, while at the opposite pole internalization and preservation of the object is desired. There is a basic conflict between the impulse to destroy the object to which some threatening subjective impulse has been ascribed, and the wish to protect the object with which the subject has identified, thus investing it with narcissistic cathexis. The ego is faced with a need to maintain inner stability in the face of structural regression with its attendant threat of loss of control and instinctual discharge. It is interesting in this regard that paranoid patients are terribly threatened by any attempt to confront them with their rage and disappointment with regard to significant objects, primary objects in particular. The paranoid position often seems calculated to preserve both these objects and the object relation. The ambivalence in the relationship is too difficult to tolerate, and the rage against the object cannot be faced. These relationships are often the important source of introjects, and the projection to others provides a way of preserving the good aspects of the object relationship. On another level, projection onto such important introjective objects provides a way of preserving the relation, even if on desperate terms.

The duality of preserving and annihilating, of introjecting and projecting, is inherent in the full spectrum of paranoid states. What appears most significant in the operation of these mechanisms is that there seems to be a close relation to situations or circumstances in which the ego has suffered, or is about to suffer, a significant loss. At such points the ego is confronted with its own inner sense of inadequacy and weakness. The mechanisms operate in the direction of preserving the inner elements that support self-esteem and its related narcissism. The complex of projection/introjection operates to rework the object relations involved so as to preserve the self in a meaningful context of relatedness. The analogue is the interplay of infantile projection/introjection in establishing the self and building its relatedness to objects. Consequently, the operation of these mechanisms cannot be regarded in isolation as a result of intrapsychic dynamisms alone, but must be seen in the larger context of the subject's relatedness to objects and his embeddedness in a social context.

While the defenses are operating in an attempt to preserve self, it is apparent that their capacity to do so is limited. The paranoid patient is under duress from within and from without. His defensive struggle is aimed at rejecting the painful and evil parts of the self and locating them outside (projection) and affiliating unto himself the fragments of relationships that can enhance his sense of self and his relatedness to the world of objects around him (introjection). But the attempt is abortive, as both projection and introjection operate in part to diminish the sense of self. Projection preserves a relation to the object of a certain distorted quality, but at the expense of loss of the projected parts of the self and compromise of the capacity to relate in ways that facilitate the growth and integration of self.

Introjection preserves the relation to the object within the ego, but in so doing creates an internalized presence that is subject to primary process influences and preserves its derivative character. The cost to the self is a persistent infringement on internal consistency and a reduction in the capacity to relate to objects more maturely. The defensive operation of introjection, therefore, attains some self-preservative compromise, but it interferes with the ego's capacity to integrate itself less in drive-derivative terms and more in terms of mature object relatedness. Introjection in its early developmental aspects allows the emerging ego to "work through" primary process types of structural organization, but in its defensive aspects tends to fix processes of internal structural formation in drive-derivative primary process types of organization, and thus prevents the emergence of more autonomous secondary process forms of ego integration (Meissner, 1970).

MELANIE KLEIN AND PROJECTION

If Freud's description provides us a starting point, our next task is to examine the contribution of Melanie Klein. Klein's position derives essentially from Freud's, but adds its own particular emphasis.

Klein's earliest thinking on projection finds its point of origin in Freud's "Beyond the Pleasure Principle" (1920). Following Freud, Klein postulated the operation of the death instinct from the beginning of life, as both opposed to and bound by libido (the life instinct). To escape annihilation by its own inner destructiveness, the organism's narcissistic or self-directed libido forces the destructive instinct outward and directs it against objects. Along with this, intrapsychic defenses are mobilized against residues of the death instinct that could not be externalized. The result is an excessive tension in the infantile ego, felt as anxiety related specifically to the death instinct, and resulting in a division in instinctual levels, setting one part against the other. These early defenses form the foundation of the nascent, infantile superego.

Formation of the superego advances when the child makes its earliest oral introjection of these same objects with their destructive projective attributes. The projected sadism is once again internalized, so that the child becomes dominated by fears of unimaginably cruel attacks both from real objects and from the new internal superego. The resulting anxiety increases the child's sadism and the wish to destroy hostile objects and thus escape their attacks. This results in a vicious circle in which the anxious impulse to destroy the object results in increased anxiety and superego severity. Excessive anxiety leads to a process of splitting in the superego and allows further displacement of destructive elements into the external world, thus decreasing the violence of intrapsychic conflicts (Klein, 1929). The displacement by projection diminishes the internal anxiety and moderates the tension of the truce between superego and id. Klein sees such mechanisms operating not only in the personification and animation of childhood play, but also in analytic transferences.

The early domination of these processes of introjection and projection by aggression and anxiety leads to a basic fear of persecuting objects, which Klein has designated as the paranoid-schizoid position. However, in addition to such persecutory fears, there is a pining for loved objects, which leads gradually to a fear of losing them. Klein (1935) describes this as the depressive position. The introjection of the loved object (now experienced as a whole object as opposed to a part-object) gives rise to concern and sorrow that the good object might be destroyed by the bad objects and their associated destructive impulses.

In order to escape the suffering connected with the depressive position, the ego may take refuge in good objects, either by a flight to a good internalized object, taking the form of an excessive belief in the benevolence and protective power of these internalized objects (which may result in severe psychotic denial), or by a flight to external good objects leading to idealizations and excessive dependence on these objects, with a corresponding weakening of the ego (Klein, 1935). Failure to resolve the dilemmas of the infantile depressive position may result in depression, mania, or paranoia. Obsessional, manic, or paranoid defenses serve the purpose of enabling the individual to escape depressive pain. They may be mobilized pathologically in the failure to experience mourning, but are regarded by Klein as an essential part of normal development as well.

Consequently, Klein's elaboration of Freud's notion of projection shifts it from the level of functioning as a mechanism of pathological symptom formation to a central process of psychic development generally, in the sense that it makes a central contribution to personality development and, in addition, serves to deal defensively with excessive degrees of aggression and anxiety, thus becoming a central mechanism in the development of pathogenic processes.

It might be well, for the purposes of our argument, to focus particularly on the emphasis given to projection in Klein's formulation. Rather than regarding it as a mechanism of defense against painful internal stimuli or a device for attributing internal stimuli to an external source, Klein makes projection a necessary process and the point of origin for object relations. The death instinct is postulated as the driving force, and projection as the necessary mechanism for mitigating its internal destructive power. It is the death instinct, through projection, in a sense, that creates objects and the relation to them. The organism then creates powerful, destructive, and persecutory objects.

In addition, Klein's formulation signals an important methodological shift. Freud's emphasis was on mechanisms that give rise to certain symptoms; Klein places the emphasis rather on fantasy production in the articulation and formulation of these processes. The process is immediately translated into and expressed in terms of its correlative infantile fantasies of persecution, destruction, oral incorporation, devouring, expelling, etc. Consequently, the Kleinian discussion of object relations is cast not in the language of real relationship but rather in the instinctually derived language of fantasies about objects and their relation to the subject.

PROJECTIVE IDENTIFICATION

As Klein developed her ideas about projection, the emphasis on fantasy and the connection with introjection became predominant dimensions. The oral sadistic attack on the mother's breast is extended to her body in the impulse to suck, bite, scoop out, and rob her body of its good contents. The oral sadistic fantasies become bound up with greed, that is, the wish to empty the mother's body of everything good and desirable that might be in it. Introjection in Klein's usage is connected with oral incorporative fantasies.

The other impulses that play a role are those deriving from anal and urethral zones, which imply the expelling of dangerous toxic substances out of the self and into the mother. Along with these poisonous excrements, the bad and hated parts of the self are split off and projected *into* the mother—Klein insists on the "into." The projected parts not only injure but also serve to control and take possession of the object. The mother then contains the bad parts of the self thus projected, and as such—as Klein (1946) emphasizes—"she is not felt to be a separate individual but is felt to be *the* bad self" (p. 102). In this connection, Klein introduces the term projective identification: "Much of the hatred against parts of the self is now directed toward the mother. This leads to a particular form of identification which establishes the prototype of an aggressive object-relation. I suggest for these processes the term 'projective identification'" (1946, p. 102).

Projective identification thus derives from the splitting of the ego and the projection of parts of the self into others, primarily the mother and her breast. It is a fantasy of the omnipotent expulsion of bodily substances in order to control and take possession of the object. The object then is not felt to be separate, but is experienced as an aspect of the self (Klein, 1963). Klein refers to these processes as identification by projection (projective identification) and its complementary process, identification by introjection. Introjective identification starts with the child's earliest relation to the breast, even in the vampire fantasies of sucking and biting. Introjective identification is thus synonymous with the greed-based oral-sadistic introjection of the mother's breast. Thus, introjection and projection interact from the very beginning of life.

POST-KLEINIAN DEVELOPMENTS

In considering post-Kleinian developments, it seems clear that most Kleinian thinkers recognize to some degree the basically psychotic character of projective identification and acknowledge the aspects of self-fragmentation, diffusion of identity, and loss of self-object differentiation that it implies. Rosenfeld (1952), for example, describes the operation of projective identification in schizophrenic productions, including the tendency to fusion with objects. This confusion is attributed not only to fantasies of oral incorporation as an aspect of introjective identification, but also to the impulses and fantasies of penetrating into the object with the whole or a part of one's self, as in projective identification. Following Klein, Rosenfeld (1964) regards this as the most primitive form of object relation. The confusion between self and object is precisely the outcome of the operation of projective identification:

> Identification is an important factor in narcissistic object-relations. It may take place by introjection or by projection. When the object is omnipotently incorporated, the self becomes so identified with the incorporated object that all separate identity or any boundary between self and object is denied. In projective identification parts of the self omnipotently enter an object, for example, the mother, to take over certain qualities which would be experienced as desirable, and therefore claim to be the object or part-object. Identification by introjection and by projection usually occur simultaneously. [p. 333]

The result of these processes is a fundamental confusion and an incapacity to differentiate subject and object, reality and fantasy, along with an inability to differentiate the real object from its symbolic representation (Rosenfeld, 1952). When we turn to the efforts of Wilfred Bion, who has been responsible, perhaps more than anyone else, for the extension of the notion of projective identification, the same basic realization seems operative. Projective identification is exemplified as a basic mechanism in the schizophrenic process and reflects the regressive reconstitution of the paranoid-schizoid position. For Bion, as for Klein, projective identification represents an omnipotent fantasy that unwanted parts of the personality or of the internal objects (acquired by introjection) can be disowned, projected, and contained within the object into which they are projected. In consequence, parts of the ego are thus projected into the object, and the object is experienced as controlled by the projected parts and imbued with specific qualities related to those parts. In Bion's terms, when such projective identification is operating in pathological terms, the outcome is a psychotic condition with intensified envy and greed, and is reflected in the heightened operations of splitting and projection. This leads to the projection of fragmented, bizarre, and persecutory objects and a corresponding emptying out of the subject ego. Particles of ego functioning are fragmented and evacuated, and by projection come to penetrate, occupy, and engulf the real object. Correspondingly, the persecutory object comes to attack the projected part and strips it of any reality or vitality. The object thus becomes a bizarre object composed of parts of the self and parts of the object in a relationship of container and contained that strips both of any inherent vitality or meaning.

Bion extends the notion of projective identification in terms of his metaphor of the container and the contained. The metaphor is based on the image of the infant expelling destructive content into the mother, who accepts the infant's projection, contains it, and modifies it so that its destructiveness is in some degree neutralized, thus allowing for reintrojection on the part of the infant. The content of the infant's reintrojecting is made more tolerable and more potentially integrable in the extent to which it has been modified or metabolized by the good-mothering qualities of the maternal object. In this usage, projective identification comes to stand for the relationship between mother and child, and it is this relationship that is internalized to give rise to the child's cognitive apparatus. In Bion's terms, then, projective identification is a form of symbiotic relationship taking place in reciprocally beneficial ways between two persons, between a container and a contained. Consequently, projective identification becomes a metaphor, translated loosely into the terms of container and contained, which applies to almost any form of relational or cognitive phenomenon in which the common notes of relation, containment, or implication can be appealed to.

An interesting attempt to broaden the meaning of projective identification, particularly in reference to the therapeutic process, is that of Malin and Grotstein (1966). Their argument follows Kleinian lines. Projection is distinguished from projective identification in that the former is viewed solely as a mechanism for dealing with instinctual drives. This follows the early Kleinian formulation according to which aggressive or libidinal impulses are projected onto the object. But since instinctual organization and development take place in a context of object relations, the psyche can be viewed as a dynamic structure (à la Fairbairn) composed of internalized objects and part-objects cathected by drive impulses. The connection of these drive components with parts of the self (the internalized objects or so-called identifications) imply the link with internalization and justify use of the term projective identification as opposed to simple projection (of drive components only). Consequently, the authors take the position that all projection includes identification and, conversely, that all identification includes projection. They expand this notion in the following argument:

We must tentatively project out a part of our inner psychic contents in order to be receptive to the object for introjection and subsequently to form an identification with it. When we start with the projection it is necessary that there be some process of identification or internalization in general, or else we can never be aware of the projection. That is, what is projected would be lost like a satellite rocketed out of the gravitational pull of the earth. . . . A projection, of itself, seems meaningless unless the individual can retain some contact with what is projected. That contact is a type of internalization, or, loosely, an identification. [p.27]

This formulation reflects a general tendency to focus the notion of projective identification in the context of transference and countertransference interactions in the analytic setting. In these terms, the mechanisms and processes on which the phenomena of transference and countertransference and their complex interactions are based are those of projection and introjection—or, in Kleinian terms, projective or introjective identification (Fliess, 1953; Racker, 1953, 1957; Money-Kyrle, 1956; Grinberg, 1962). In the argument advanced by Malin and Grotstein (1966), all transferences and countertransferences involve, and are based on, projective identifications.

Other contributors insist on the distinction, in these contexts, between projective identification and projection as such. Jaffe (1968) points to differences in the degree of intrapsychic splitting and projective annihilation of the object as discriminating factors. Kernberg (1965) emphasizes the more regressive aspects of projective identification, especially the blurring of ego boundaries. There is room for discussing whether the phenomena in question justify talk of anything beyond the mechanisms of introjection and projection and their complex interactions.

There has also been a certain vogue in using the concept of projective identification to describe complex patterns of interacting projection and introjection within family systems. Zinner and Shapiro (1972) view projective identification as bridging the gap between individual dynamics and social interaction within the family system. They write:

Projective identification is an activity of the ego which, among its effects, modifies perception of the object and, in a reciprocal fashion, alters the image of the self. These conjoined changes in perception influence and may, in fact, govern behavior of the self toward the object. Thus projective identification provides an important conceptual bridge between an individual and interpersonal psychology, since our awareness of the mechanisms permits us to understand specific interactions *among* persons in terms of specific dynamic conflicts occurring *within* individuals. [p. 523]

Implicit in this view of projective identification as operating within family systems is an interactional perspective; that is, the projective and identificatory components are not referred to single individuals, as interacting intrapsychic components, but rather are located in the interaction between two or more individuals. The interaction in this case is presumed to include (a) a projection from the subject; (b) an introjection on the part of the other, who receives and internalizes the content of the projection; (c) a counterprojection from the other onto the original subjects; (d) a subsequent introjection on the part of the subject of what has been correspondingly projected onto him; (e) a subjective perception of the object, as if the object contained parts of the subject's own personality; (f) an ability on the part of the subject to elicit behaviors, attitudes, or feelings in the other that conform to the subject's projection; and, finally, (g) a frequent collusion among the participants in such close, emotionally involved relationships in order to maintain mutual projections and their corresponding introjective organizations (Zinner and Shapiro, 1972; Meissner, 1978a, 1978b). In some accounts, presumably Kleinian, the projections in this sequence are equivalent to the fantasy of expelling part of the self into another, such that the expelled part takes over the other and induces the other to respond in terms of the dictates of the projection (Ogden, 1979). In any case, the process has become interactive and interpersonal.

CONCLUSION

This has been a long and tortuous odyssey that has led in the direction of increasing complexity and diffusion of concepts. From Freud's original formulation of simple projection to the more recent elaborations of the notion of projective identification, there has occurred a gradual broadening and a confusing proliferation of implications in our attempts to understand the complexities of the interactions between internalizations and externalizations. The simple defense mechanism identified by Freud was first linked conceptually and functionally with the structure of internalizations. In the hands of Melanie Klein these notions were transformed doubly: on the one hand, from issues of specific conflict and defense into aspects of intrapsychic development and the developmental process, and, on the other, from forms of structural organization into a metapsychology of fantasy.

The shift from the analysis of separate mechanisms (projection, introjection) to the concept of projective identification tended to compound these separately interactive components into a single complex conceptualization that was originally cast in terms of the operation of fantasy systems. The early implications of this approach pointed to the role of psychotic fantasies, with connotations of loss of reality testing and degrees of self-object de-differentiation. Later extrapolations of this notion have broadened the application of projective identification to include wider ranging, nonpsychotic expressions, and have tended to shift attention from intrapsychic and fantasy-based aspects to the complex contexts of human interaction, in which reciprocally engaged processes of internalization and externalization occurring between and among subjects are at issue. The question that confronts us, it seems to me, is whether this theoretical development has served to deepen our understanding of the complexity of human mental processes and interactions, or whether it has served only to engender terminological and conceptual confusion, thus posing a barrier to more effective therapy.

It may help for purposes of discussion, at least to the extent of providing a visible target, for me to state my own conclusions based on this extensive review of the literature on projective identification and my own clinical experience. I can summarize my present view in the following points:

1. There is a legitimate place for the term projective identification, but its scope is quite limited. I advocate a return to the original sense of the term as proposed by Melanie Klein. She intended it to describe an intrapsychic mechanism that occurs as part of a psychotic process, in which the self or some part of the self is projected into the object and in which the self becomes identified with the object so modified. Since the process remains intrapsychic, it would presumably be more accurate to speak here of projection into the object *representation*.

In any case, the process involves loss of self-object differentiation, diffusion of ego boundaries, and absorption of the self, or that part of the self that is projected, into the object. Correspondingly, the self loses its sense of independent existence. Consequently, projective identification in this sense could be viewed as the form of externalization that corresponds to the process of incorporation as a form of internalization. In incorporation the object is internalized in such a fashion that the object is assimilated to the subject and thus loses its separate status as an independent object. This too should be regarded as a psychotic process (Meissner, 1981).

2. An important distinction that comes into play in this regard is that between process and fantasy. When we speak of projective identification, are we referring to a mental process as a part of the operative structure of the mind, or are we addressing a phenomenon of fantasy. If the patient speaks in terms of a fantasy that he is able to put his thoughts into other people's heads and thus control their minds, we do not as yet have sufficient ground to regard what he is describing as a process occurring in his mind. It is no more than a fantasy. If the patient begins to act as though he were able to put thoughts in others' minds and as though he were in consequence able to control their minds and actions, then we might be on better footing for drawing a conclusion that an actual mental process is involved.

The distinction in question is even clearer in the case of internalizations. These mental processes are invariably connected with fantasies of incorporation. The fantasy may be to some degree unconscious, but it is a constant feature of any internalization. However, the process of internalization is not equivalent to the fantasy. Patients in the terminal phase of analytic work often experience meaningful, constructive, and structure-enhancing identifications that are selective, organized in secondary process terms, and facilitative of a sense of autonomous self-integration (Meissner, 1981). Such internalizations are clearly not based on primitive incorporations, but they may be (and often are) associated with oral incorporative fantasies.

Perhaps this distinction draws a line between the Kleinian viewpoint and analytic orientations that prefer to adhere more closely to the natural science model. The latter approach treats matters of fantasy and metaphor as content and looks for other data to determine the nature of the mental processes that produce and modify such content.

3. An important distinction that needs to be kept in the foreground of any discussion of projective identification is the distinction between a one-body context and a two-or-more-body context. There is a radical difference in projective identification as it occurs in the two contexts. In the one-body context, both the projection and the identification take place in one mind: the projection takes place in relation to the subject's own object representation, and the ensuing identification takes place entirely as an intrapsychic event. In the two-or-more-body context, the projection takes place in one mind while the identification(s) take place in

other minds. Because of the correlative nature of the processes involved, I prefer to regard the internalizations in question as introjections (Meissner, 1981).

Such correlative and interlocking projections and introjections occur in any transference-countertransference situation, as we have noted. They occur also in group situations. But in whatever context, there are separate processes taking place in different heads. Any attempt to extend the usage from the one-body context to the more-than-one-body context can only sow the seeds of confusion and obfuscation.

A further point should be made in this regard. Some authors attempt to distinguish projection and projective identification on the basis that the latter carries with it a propensity to draw the object of the projection into a position of responding to the implicit demand of the projection and in complementary fashion internalizing the projective elements. This distinction strikes me as spurious. Such complementary pulls are at work in all projections occurring in an interpersonal context; no inherently different mechanism is involved. There is only the difference that the projection is operating in an interpersonal field and within that field has its inevitable consequences, one of which is to create emotional pressures to draw the object into compliance with the projection and to reinforce it. In these interpersonal contexts, it seems simpler and more correct to speak of patterns of projection and introjection. The term projective identification obscures more than it reveals.

APPENDIX: CLINICAL EXAMPLES

The following clinical examples are appended for purposes of discussion. I have selected the clinical material, not with an eye to providing a catalogue of forms of projective identification, but to make a major point: that each of the examples might be categorized as involving projective identification, but that each can easily and more simply be regarded as involving no more than projections and introjections of varying quality and complexity. I would like to give three examples of the interplay of introjective and projective processes as they operate in different contexts and different types of personality structure.

1. The first example is that of a young man in his late twenties, whose personality structure was quite primitive, severely borderline (psychotic character), and organized in paranoid fashion. I will focus on the phenomenology of the patient's introjective configuration and its relation to paranoid manifestations.

The patient suffered from ideas of reference and persecution. He imagined as he walked down the street that the people passing him were staring at him, thinking him a piece of good-for-nothing scum, the lowest and the most contemptible and inferior of human beings, despising him, hating him, and even wanting to kill him. At times, these delusions would reach the point of an overwhelming fear that as he strolled along someone would suddenly turn on him, pull out a gun or knife, and shoot or stab him to death. This fear would become so overwhelming that he had actually to run from the street and find an escape. For example, on one occasion the patient ventured forth to buy a new suit and went to a large department store. As he came through the front door of the store, he was suddenly overwhelmed with a terrifying fear that armed guards were posted along the balcony of the store, submachine guns trained on him and about to kill him. He turned on his heels and ran from the store in panic. I would take these experiences as expressing the projection of the aspects of the patient's own unresolved aggressive and destructive impulses.

But there was another side to this. At other points in his treatment the patient would describe himself as walking down the street, looking about at the people who passed by and feeling a powerful sense of contempt and hatred for them; he would even experience fantasies of carrying a submachine gun under his coat and suddenly pulling it out in the middle of a crowded thoroughfare and spraying everyone in sight with a sudden and deadly hail of bullets. He had a special hatred for establishment institutions, particularly large corporations (his father had worked as a highly placed executive in one of these). At times he would recount passing the office buildings of such corporations and imagining himself hurling a Molotov cocktail or an explosive charge through the front windows. At such fantasies, the patient would feel a sense of elatedness and power, a feeling that he could bring even great corporations and powerful institutions to their knees.

These experiences convey a sense of the powerful interplay between aggressively derived introjects and their corresponding projections. In these examples, the patient plays out the interrelationship between the aggressor introject and the victim introject. In the first set of instances, he becomes the powerless, helpless, attacked, and persecuted victim, while the persecuting and attacking forces about him are attributed strength, power, and destructive hostility. In the later contexts, however, this situation is reversed, as the elements of the aggressor introject come to dominate the patient's experience of himself, and the objects of his powerful and destructive attacks become the helpless and powerless victims, the projective representatives of his own sense of vulnerability, impotence, and victimization.

The same patient played out the dialectic of introjection and projection around narcissistic issues as well. At times, the sense of narcissistic inferiority dominated his self-awareness, and was matched by the projected superiority of those around him. At such times, the patient would be overwhelmed by a sense of shame and worthlessness, a feeling that he was the lowest of the low, a worm and no man, and that no one could know him or have anything to do with him and not have utter contempt for him, despising him as he despised himself. In his paranoid fashion he would be convinced that the people who crossed his path did in fact harbor such feelings of contempt. Even in this experience the patient reveals the polarities of pathogenic narcissistic introjection. Aspects of the inferior narcissistic introjection are expressed in the feelings of shame and diminished self-esteem, while the attitudes of critical superiority and contempt reflect the narcissistic configuration of superiority. This superiority is projected to external objects even as the patient experiences his own self-devaluation.

The opposite side of the narcissistic coin was expressed at points at which the patient would angrily and contemptuously revile public figures or important academic or business representatives, devaluing their attainments, criticizing their intelligence, and holding them up to ridicule, with the repeated claim that he was better read and had a more penetrating and encompassing understanding than these powerful and influential individuals. Again, the dialectic of narcissistic extremes, both positive and negative, were played out in terms of the patient's projections and corresponding internalizations.

2. The second case I will describe is that of a woman in her mid-thirties who evinced a depressive-masochistic character. This woman came into treatment for chronic and recurrently exacerbated depression. It turned out that she was immersed in a severely sadomasochistic marriage in which she self-sacrificingly bent every effort, even to the extremes of self-denial, to gain some sense of approval from her husband. This enterprise he continually frustrated, demeaning her and showing a callous disregard for her needs and wishes. In the face of overwhelming evidence to the contrary, she stoutly maintained the perception that he was in fact a kind, generous, and good man, and that she herself was inadequate, undeserving of his good graces, and even evil. She saw herself as helpless and powerless, and considered her only function in the marriage to be that of the dutiful wife whose job it was to cater to her powerful and perfect

husband's every whim. Even after she was able to appreciate the neurotic character of her posture and the distorted aspects of the relationship, and even after she had effectively filed for divorce, she would approach any negotiation or contact with her former husband with a sense of dread. In their dealings over the custody of the children she maintained the conviction that he was the powerful one, who had on his side all the resources of the law, position, and wealth, while she herself felt acutely a sense of her inadequacy as a parent, her lack of resources, and her inability to deal with his demands and manipulations. As she saw it, she had no recourse but to keep her mouth shut and submit to whatever he saw fit to impose on her.

This kind of pathology, familiar to all clinicians, shows how the patterning of the victim introject and the corresponding aggressor introject play themselves out in this type of personality organization. Not only did the patient experience herself in terms of the victim introject, but her projection of the aggressive components onto her husband turned him into an incomparably powerful, influential, and potentially destructive figure. Obviously, my patient was dealing with rather deep-seated conflicts over aggression, which did not allow her to assume a more assertive and aggressive posture but rather required that her aggressive impulses be displaced to an external object, thus allowing her to defensively maintain her own sense of vulnerability and victimization—an intrapsychic configuration that ruled out of court and out of mind any effective exercise of aggression.

The question before us is whether this complex interaction of externalization and internalization merits the title of projective identification. I would contend that no more is involved here than identifiable projections meshing with and interlocking with corresponding introjections. My patient's projection of her aggressive components onto her husband were matched by his introjection of aggression in his own right, so that they played out the drama of aggressor and victim. The concept of projective identification does nothing to clarify our clinical understanding of this process, and only adds conceptual confusion and obscurity.

3. My last example is that of a young businessman in his thirties, who came into analysis because of continuing difficulties in interpersonal relationships, particularly an inability to get along with authority figures. The patient turned out to be a quite analyzable narcissistic personality, whose interaction in the psychoanalytic situation manifests the interplay of introjective and projective elements in the transference.

The patient had grown up in a family in which his father had been a rather violent and brutal figure, often coming home drunk and beating his wife, as well as terrorizing the children. These episodes were quite regular in the patient's childhood, and often culminated in violent scenes of physical abuse, the breaking of furniture, and mother and children being driven out of the house and into the streets. The patient's mother was long-suffering and endured the brutality of the father in a self-effacing manner, placing the integrity of the family ahead of any wishes to escape from a tyrannical and abusive husband.

For many months at the beginning of his analysis, my patient effected a demeanor that was submissive and conforming, never showing the least sign of irritation or objection. He would come into my office with eyes cast down submissively, never looking at me directly, never raising his eyes from the floor. In the analysis he was exceedingly compliant, accepting without question any directive or suggestion I might make. As the analysis progressed, this remarkable lack of even an inkling of assertion, of aggressiveness, or of resentful or hostile feelings toward the analyst became increasingly evident. It gradually emerged that, as he approached my office and entered it, he was overwhelmed with feelings of anxiety and fear, experiencing me as a powerful, even magical, figure who would tolerate him only if he were submissive and compliant in the extreme. He spoke of his seeing me as though I were a powerful lion or tiger and he, correspondingly, a frightened and timorous little mouse.

The origins of these transference feelings in his relationship to his father were quite transparent, but it was not until later in the analytic work that the aggressive aspects of the introjective configuration came into focus. In relation to me and to other authority figures, the patient adopted the same submissive and conforming attitude. However, as he began to talk about his relationship to his wife, it became clear that when he came home from work in the evening and walked through the front door of his house, he changed from the timorous little mouse into the raging tiger. He would criticize and verbally abuse his wife for the least failing, the least shortcoming in her running of the house. He demanded that when he got home she have a drink ready for him, and that within a short period of time they be ready to sit down to a well-prepared and piping hot meal. He was extremely demanding and perfectionistic about what he would eat and how he wanted it prepared. When I commented that this peremptory and tyrannical behavior contrasted with his submissive demeanor outside the home, he responded that this way of behaving was very like his father's. If what his mother put on the table was not exactly to her husband's liking, he would take the dish and smash it to the floor, expecting her to clean it up. He would then fly into one of his terrible rages.

This aspect of the patient's behavior was tied in with his narcissistic dynamics, and played out his sense of entitlement, of specialness, his feeling that he deserved special consideration and service from his wife. To keep the focus on the interplay of the aggressor and victim configurations, it is clear that in his relationships with authority figures he retreated to the submissive stance dictated by the victim introject. Correspondingly, aggressive components were projected to these external figures, so that they were seen as excessively powerful, destructive, and threatening. By the same token, when the patient got home the tables were turned, not only literally but intrapsychically. He then became the aggressor and his wife the impotent victim, whose only recourse was to submit to his tyrannical demands. Thus, both sides of the introjective configurations were played out.

The same dynamics were played out in the transference. He not only saw me as powerful and threatening, but behaved in such a way as to draw me into such a position. His superficiality and withholding of meaningful analytic material were masked by a submissive and compliant style. There was a constant invitation for me to intervene, to take over, to direct the flow of material, to intrude by asking about important relationships, dreams, trying to elicit associations, and so on. There was a subtle vacuum created in the analytic space that was calculated to draw me into the position of the knowing, controlling, and powerful wizard-analyst. But behind the facade of compliance was a defiant challenge, a counterwill to defeat me, to prove me inadequate, to frustrate the goals of the analytic process, to make himself the ultimate victor and me the impotent, frustrated, and vanquished shadow that he felt himself to be.

Should we call this projective indentification? Projection, yes. And the pressure I felt, and the degree to which I found myself experiencing frustration and impatience, even being drawn into a more active, directive stance from time to time, reflected a process of internalization in me. Moreover, it was influenced and elicited by the patient's projection. I would hesitate to call it an identification for reasons I have discussed. It would be more accurate to call it an introjection. The interplay of transference projection and countertransference introjection are two separate processes, linked by affective connections, but nonetheless separate and independent, and taking place in two different agents. These processes have no connection with the sense of projective identification identifiable in an intrapsychic (one-body) context. Applying the term projective identification adds nothing to our understanding and serves only to confuse.

Chapter 4

Discussion of W. W. Meissner's Paper

Joseph Sandler   Dr. Meissner has given us a most interesting paper with much food for thought. He has emphasized the role of projective and introjective mechanisms in psychic development, and the parts they play in establishing the difference between inner and outer, between self and object. Throughout he has stressed the developmental point of view, and has considered a number of important topics, including the role of introjection in superego formation. It is of particular interest that throughout his presentation it is demanded of us that we take into account the idea of an interaction between self and object. Such interaction can be intrapsychic or interpersonal and is aimed at establishing some sort of inner balance. It is not considered simply an expression of drive impulses, in the way in which self-object interactions were viewed in the past. Dr. Meissner has made a distinction between the early *developmental* role of projection and the *defensive* projection that can occur only when the boundary between self and object has been established. In the latter, the boundary is a necessary condition for the projection to be effective.

As far as projective identification is concerned, Dr. Meissner has said very clearly that he now finds the concept far too broad to be useful. I suspect that many will disagree with him, and we may legitimately ask what he would substitute for the concept. Is it enough to say that the phenomena it covers are but a combination of projective and introjective mechanisms? There is also the question of whether projective identification is a psychotic mechanism.

In listening to Dr. Meissner I felt that it might be useful to have some clarification with regard to the distinction between identification and introjection. I, for one, was not very happy about the broad use of "introjection" to refer to a number of very different processes. One clear

51

use of the term in Dr. Meissner's paper was to refer to what I would call identification, a process in which there is a change in the self-representation on the basis of an aspect of an object representation. In a sense, it could be said that an object "is taken into" the self. But there is also the notion of introjection as the setting up of an internal companion, so to speak, with whom one can have a dialogue but who is not a part of one's self-representation. The introject is then more of a back-seat driver, someone who tells one what to do—in either a friendly or an unfriendly fashion—and with whom one can have an unconscious interchange, just as one might have a conscious one with a real external object. The notion of internal object relationships is crucial here, and unless one clarifies the distinction between internalization into the self-representation and internalization into the object aspects of the internal world—the introjects—we may get into difficulties. I would very much like to hear Dr. Meissner's views on that. This point leads us to a notion of a possible identification with the introject as well as with the external object, but this is not a point I want to labor at the moment.

Some of us may have questions about the effect of externalizations on the other person, and about the way in which we can simultaneously identify with and yet dissociate ourselves from some aspect of the self that has been externalized onto or into another person. I refer, of course, in this last point, to the mechanism of projective identification.

W. W. Meissner. I should like to respond to Dr. Sandler's comments, which I think are very relevant. I would preface my response by remarking that we all engage in this very difficult area in very personal ways. We are concerned with the complicated issue of what is implied in the commerce between the internal development of our own psychic life and the experience that we have of the world around us and the people in it. Within this area the elaborate terminology that has developed represents a variety of attempts to come to terms, from different theoretical perspectives, with that very complex interaction, and to begin to make some sense out of it—particularly, to make sense of it in ways that relate to our psychoanalytic concerns.

If, when presented with that smorgasbord of concepts, we attempted to take something of everything, we would get a bad case of indigestion. The only way we will find nourishment in this business is to be rather selective, and to pick and choose in terms of what tastes good to us. This means that one cannot claim that there is any absolute priority or superiority in any of these various approaches. It is all very subjective. There is an old scholastic maxim that says *de gustibus non est disputandum* (one cannot argue about tastes). That is the situation we are up against. What we should be able to do, I think, in a discussion of this nature, is to get a sense from the various presentations of their advantages and disadvantages, of the usefulness and limitations of any particular approach to these difficult notions.

I have commented that I don't find the notion of projective identification very useful. Well, that is a personal appraisal. One of the reasons I have not found it useful is perhaps that I have not dealt with the kind of patients, by and large, in whom projective identification is said to be frequently encountered. But perhaps that implies that I have scrapped my notion of projective identification, so it is a question not of replacing it with something else, but rather of finding the locale and focus within which the concept of projective identification makes sense. Now, I do think that the early Kleinian usage of projective identification makes sense. It describes something I have experienced with psychotic patients, and when I read the clinical descriptions of the application of the projective identification concept in this way it makes perfectly good sense to me. What does not make such good sense is the application of the idea to other phenomena, where I am not at all sure there are the same implications or even the same kinds of descriptive phenomenology. This reflects a problem in regard to analytic concepts, and here I have the notion of a "diffusion quotient." One can take almost any analytic concept, and notice that it starts with a fairly discrete and focused application in terms of some aspect of the clinical phenomena. At the beginning it is useful and enlightening in that context, but before one can blink one's eyes it is as if we have a large pile of sand, which is piled higher and higher until it loses the force that has kept it together. It is diffused over a vast terrain of allied phenomena, and one begins to lose any sense of its precision or exactness. So when we use the term projective identification, for example, we are talking about something that is in some sense the same, but also in some sense different. There has to be a cut-off point, to my mind, where the kind of analogous diffusion of the concept becomes less than productive. This is the point at which it has begun to become applied in too vast a way to allow us to understand complex phenomena. In the long run, attempts to be more precise and more exact in the use of concepts might be more productive, more insightful, and more helpful, even within the clinical context. So when I think about projective identification my view of it is much closer to the original Kleinian one.

There is another complex issue here. What I am looking for in this area does not have to do with content or fantasy. It has to do with *process*.

There is a very special emphasis here which is characteristic of the mainstream of American psychoanalytic thinking in that it is much more concerned with issues of understanding the processes and the mechanisms that enter psychic manifestations than with the fantasies involved. Historically, this is probably due to the influence of the ego psychology school of Heinz Hartmann, David Rapaport, and Ernst Kris, although the whole tendency has gone well beyond their influence, I think. In that context content is not immediately translatable into intrapsychic mechanisms or processes. So when we talk of projective identification it is not enough to refer to a fantasy of placing a part of the self into an object. One has to go further and find evidence for a process which would have that kind of implication. So one would not be satisfied in that conceptual context that projective identification has occurred if the patient simply reports material that can be understood as reflecting a fantasy in which he regards some part of himself as embedded in another object. One would want to see concrete data that suggest that indeed that process has taken place. One would have to find evidence of the process's having occurred, and could not presume that its existence is entailed by that of the fantasy.

The situation is similar with incorporation. Incorporation in fantasy is probably related to all internalization processes. If we go back to the early literature on internalization, much of it is expressed in terms of oral incorporation. But again, we can ask about what is being expressed when that kind of material is produced in an analysis or other therapeutic situation. Is it simply a fantasy, or is there a mechanism and a process of incorporation that goes along with it that we can put our finger on? One context where this comes into play with distinct clarity is in the termination phase—I am speaking of relatively healthy patients now—when patients will actually talk about incorporating the analyst, devouring the analyst, wanting to take the analyst into themselves, and there is a very oral connotation in the content. But what is in fact going on is a much more sophisticated process of internalization that cannot be equated with primitive oral material. It is a quite different kind of process, and when one tries to identify it it is not the same as the fantasy. One would not say in that context that the patient *is* incorporating. One would say that the patient has a fantasy of incorporation, but that fantasy incorporation is attendant on a process of an entirely different order, one that can be defined quite discretely in metapsychological terms.

Wolfgang Berner (Austria). I have a question concerning the connection between identification and projection. It refers to a special case of a pedophilic patient who could simultaneously be himself and the little boy he once was. In the role of the little boy he lived out and acted out a fantasy connecting him with his mother, and in this he projected and also introjected both parts of himself. He projected aspects of his own self into the boy and into himself. I think that in such cases of pedophilic activity one can see a greater connection between introjection and projection than in psychotic cases. Would you see this in the same way? I would add that one of the points the man sought in little boys was that they should be braver than he was, more provoking, in the same way as his mother provoked him when he was a little boy. The activities he gratified with the boys were that he tried to touch their genitals with his fingers, and then experienced a very tender feeling toward them.

W. W. Meissner.   I want to make it clear that I am not saying that if one can identify projections and introjections that this has any diagnostic implication. Projections and introjections of various kinds take place up and down the broad spectrum of human experience. We all do our share of projecting and introjecting, and the operation of these mechanisms is an extremely important part of what happens in the analytic situation. And it is not just on the part of the patient that these mechanisms enter into the common space that evolves where the transference seems to flourish. It is on the part of both participants, and they are both engaged in a kind of introjective-projective dance, if you will, that plays itself out and shapes not only the emergence of the transference but how the transference evolves within the analytic setting and is gradually resolved. So I won't point to any specific diagnostic connotations that one can identify with these patterns. I wonder, in the case you are describing, just how the patient experiences himself in these relationships. Does he experience himself as a sort of controlling or powerful person? What is the quality of that?

Wolfgang Berner.   What struck me most was that it was impossible to discover while analyzing this patient whether he was touching himself or another object. Self and object were connected in such a way that it wasn't possible to find the boundary. Was he relating to another object or to himself?

W. W. Meissner.   So it seems there was some splitting and confusion in his representations of himself and of the object. Well, that would be a much more primitive process, not necessarily related simply to the projective components, but obviously involving other aspects that would have to do with inner fragmentation. The dissociating off of this part of his experience is somehow alien to the inner sense of self.

Paulina Kernberg (USA).   My two questions relate in a way to the

questions that Dr. Sandler asked initially, and refer to the relation between internalization and the representations of self and object. I want to
ask whether Dr. Meissner makes any differentiation between representations of self and object on the one hand, and self- and object images on the
other. I ask this because I think there is a potential here for some
clarification of what we are talking about. My second question relates to
externalization onto another person, and here I would like to bring up
what I consider to be projective identification in the countertransference
in the case described by Dr. Meissner. I don't know whether you were the
analyst or the supervisor, but in the second case, that of the masochistic
woman, all of us heard your comments about the husband of the patient
being a really mean person, and you talked about it with a lot of feeling. I
thought this would be a potentially good illustration of the effects of
externalization on the other person. So then the other person feels very
strongly about it, and may miss what the patient's contribution to the
process is. This may affect the psychoanalytic technique or the supervisory
capacity, if one is the supervisor.

   Anne-Marie Sandler (Israel/U.K.). I also wanted to ask a simple
question, which perhaps ties in with what Paulina Kernberg has asked, but
for me it links with the third clinical case, the man who is alternately
aggressor and victim. You described how he comes into the consulting
room, and it seemed to me that entering in a very compliant way, not
looking at the analyst but rather at his shoes, appearing to be so shy and so
mouselike that he cannot even look the analyst in the eye, would make
the analyst feel many things. I, for one, would be very disturbed if my
patient looked at my feet all the time. I would like him to be able to look at
me, and I have no doubt that a patient of the sort described would arouse
many emotions in me as reactions to his behavior. I would find it very
important to find out the central features in the fantasy of this patient
which would enter into the content of his fantasies of being a victim,
whatever these fantasies may be. There is another point, which I thought
was very clearly stated by Dr. Meissner and which I found very interesting.
Let us take the same patient again. We could easily say that the man had
extremely aggressive impulses which he could not accept inside him, or
very aggressive introjects that he projected outward so the world outside
became a very aggressive, dangerous place and he became a victim. At
times he switched roles. But I think we cannot forget either that this man
must also have strong loving impulses and longings, and that his switching
from being the victim to being the aggressor has an accompanying fantasy
of being loved. He can in fact, through some of his behavior, make the

object react in a way that gets him at least *some* attention, if not the kind of love that *we* might call love. I would add that in order to complete the description of what goes on with this patient, who is obviously very rich in his imaginative life, we have to take into account what he does to the analyst, as well as the knowledge that he is very related to the world around him; and in this relationship he also maintains a loving part of himself.

Otto Kernberg.   First I want to thank Dr. Meissner for his comprehensive presentation of very complex concepts. I have some minor questions regarding specific aspects of the presentation, and then I have a major one. As far as the minor ones are concerned, I want to say, just as a point of clarification, that I believe that Dr. Meissner's comments about Klein and Bion do not at certain points quite correspond to their views. For example, you say that what Melanie Klein describes as the depressive position involves a pining for loved objects leading to a fear of losing them. It seems to me that your formulation neglects an important aspect, namely, that the depressive position represents a fear about the loss of the good internalized object threatened by internal bad objects. That is different from just pining for good objects. It is a consequence of the capacity to contain inside both good and bad objects, and therefore a fear for the survival of the good ones attacked from the inside. This is in contrast to the paranoid-schizoid position, in which the fear is over one's own survival when attacked by external persecutors.

A further point relates to your statement that Klein makes projection a necessary process and the point of origin for object relations. This also does not do her justice. She says at several points that the early ego has a number of simultaneous functions. It is the seat of anxiety, it develops object relations, and it uses projection and introjection as the very earliest mechanisms for dealing with them. For Melanie Klein the origin of object relations resides in both introjection and projection, not in projection alone.

We come now to Bion. You say that the outcome of pathological projective identification is intensified envy and greed, and is reflected in hate as well as in splitting and projection. I think that this reverses the order of the operative factors. If I understand Bion correctly, when there is intense aggression that the infant cannot handle, there is then an activation of splitting which becomes pathologically excessive—really, to the extent of fragmentation—a form of pathological splitting and violent expulsion of the fragmented aspects of intolerable aggressive internalized objects. It is that violent projection of minute fragments onto an object which creates bizarre objects. It is not that the persecutory object comes to attack the projected part, stripping it of any reality. On the contrary, it is these bizarre objects that explode or destroy the external object so that the danger arises from the effect of the bad parts having been projected outside.

Turning now to what are perhaps more major issues, I think that Dr. Meissner is right that we have to be careful when we let a concept loose and allow it to expand into ten different meanings. If I understand him correctly he is against that. But one can raise a basic methodological argument in opposition to the proposal to eliminate the concept of projective identification and to call everything either projection or introjection. If we do this we end up with so many meanings tucked under the two terms of projection and introjection that *they* lose any specific meaning. My concern, then, is that when I hear the terms introjection and projection as Dr. Meissner uses them, I find multiple meanings in them. Let me illustrate this. What do we take in when we take in anything as part of the process of relating to somebody else? Do we take in another person and put it into some place in our mind? Or do we take in an object relation? I think that the essential concept in object relations theory is that what is internalized is both the self and the object in interaction—I refer here to self-representation and object representation. If I then come back to Joseph Sandler's point, namely that what is taken in may be taken in as part of an internal object that is loved, then perhaps it is taken in as part of an internal object that motivates a modification of the self, and this is added to secondary identification of the self with the object. What is taken in may also be something which is forced upon the individual, and is conflictual and split off from other aspects of the personality. In the case of the man who had grandiose aspects to himself, he became like his father, but in obviously conflictual ways which have been distorted away from other aspects of himself. By the same token, if we now go to projection, is the attribution of good things about ourselves to someone else the same process as the attribution to the other of something unacceptable that we cannot tolerate, that we put outside ourselves in order to free ourselves from it? Is that the same as when we put something out onto the object but can't let go of it and have to control the object? Regardless of the definitions that one uses for introjection, introjective identification, projection, or projective identification, one of the advantages of these concepts is that they may capture more specific aspects of the complex process than projection or introjection alone. I want to plead for keeping a richer terminology to take care of specific clinical phenomena that differ from each other, and I think that in Dr. Meissner's metaphor of the spreading grains of sand there might be support for what I am saying.

Rivka Eifermann (Israel). Dr. Meissner, I want to go back to your paper and start on the basis of accepting what you have said. I was particularly interested in your description of the early development of projection and introjection, and your emphasis on the normal development of these processes. This is something you also pointed out with regard to the development of the superego, and their reappearance in adolescence and in the process of mourning. In regard to mourning you pointed out that the process was analogous to the interplay of infantile projection and introjection. So obviously there is a rich development in the meaning of the concepts and also in what happens to the self as it develops, and my feeling is that this is not sufficiently specified in work on these concepts. I miss in your paper a discussion of what the normal development is. I feel that you placed much more emphasis on the pathological, and in your cases did not relate your own countertransference responses to the normal development of projection and introjection.

Leslie Sohn (U.K.). I want to talk about my taste, because Dr. Meissner spoke about everybody according to his taste. I am a Kleinian training analyst from London, and therefore I have a specific taste for the clinical material as it was presented. What I cannot understand, for example, is how you know, Dr. Meissner, that the third patient's father was a brutal man. You haven't seen an X ray, nor have you seen a photograph. You simply have material. When you say, as you did in regard to the first case, that the transference was extremely rich, then you have to tell us about how you decided about the differentiation between projection and introjection in the case. You also have to explain to us how such a man, with such a bizarre set of fantasies, could actually introject. You speak as if introjection is a perfectly reasonable process, as easy as breathing. In regard to a patient with that degree of pathology I have great difficulty in accepting the idea of his ability to introject. In the second case you speak of the pathology of the lady, and you mention that you said to her that it was quite obvious that she was putting herself into extreme danger. But in terms of the transference, who are you, who are you conceived as, and did you produce her divorce by replacing the man who was bullying her? How did she develop that degree of character structure necessary to make the differentiation, to take upon herself the separation? Or was she simply split into your patient, a divorced woman, and the husband's chattel? Similarly, with the third case, I would like to know what he projected into the ground, and to know what your feet felt like, because clearly you have not told us what it felt like to be that man's analyst. As far as I can see, you have shown us that you have had at least three patients in which projective identification played very profound roles.

Joseph Sandler. Of course, this still leaves us with the problem of what each of us means by projective identification, and I hope that will be clearer as we go along. Certainly it means a great many confusing things to Dr. Meissner, so that he prefers not to use the term. Others of us use it in our own peculiar ways. As Dr. Sohn introduced the question of taste, I'd like to continue with the theme of *de gustibus*. When he and I were young analysts in London more than thirty years ago, we had very strong tastes and they corresponded to the groups we were trained in. If we digested something from another group, we had, as Dr. Meissner would put it, a bad case of indigestion. But in the course of the years I think we have developed rather cast-iron stomachs, and have been able to enjoy, to masticate and ruminate on, and to digest some of the things we have taken in from each other. This takes me to the point I want to make, and that is to the distinction which Dr. Meissner has made in the course of the discussion between mechanism and content. Now it was certainly not my taste in my psychoanalytic youth to think of mental mechanisms as fantasies. I found it, and on a theoretical level still do find it, difficult to accept that mechanisms are fantasies. But on the other hand, the Kleinians find it difficult to accept that mechanisms, as well as structures and apparatuses, are anything other than the product of that peculiar brand of ego psychology which has been produced in the United States under the influence of the New York Psychoanalytic Society. Nowadays my view would be that it really doesn't matter very much, and that we have to ask ourselves what others *mean* when they put things in their peculiar way. Neither the very concrete formulations of our Kleinian colleagues nor the very mechanistic ones of the ego psychologists should obscure the fact that the people involved are not fools. They are relating to something which is important in their clinical experience.

Turning to projective identification and to Dr. Meissner's comments in the discussion, I think that it is useful when one is dealing with the very concrete notion of putting something into somebody else to divide the process into two steps. One could say that in the unconscious fantasy of the individual—I mean the here-and-now unconscious fantasy—there is a process of getting rid of some aspect of the self or of an internal object representation, a process which is imagined very concretely in fantasy. A fantasy is created in which something is forced into another person—for example, an idealized aspect of the self. You all remember that wonderful cartoon of the woman shouting in the park "Help, help, my son the doctor is drowning." The woman obviously lived through her son, who represented ambitions of her own, and I think we have to assume that she had an effect on her son and pushed him into medical school even if she didn't actually push him into the pond. Now it is not enough to speak of that in terms of projection and introjection. We need something else as well. What I have described is what I think is the first step in projective identification, namely the construction of the unconscious fantasy (a preconscious fantasy, or a fantasy of the "adult part of the patient's self"), but more is needed. We have to add something that we can call actualization or manipulation or provocation or control of others, or something else of that sort, which is part of the whole range of the things we do to other people. We know how we constantly try to put things outside ourselves, to actualize, to reify, to make real the unconscious fantasy that involves the very concrete processes I have referred to. So it is not just a question of contrasting content or fantasy with mechanism. One performs all sorts of manipulations in fantasy first, and the mechanism involved in this is the mechanism of fantasying. But this is not enough because the projections into others do not travel through the air like the vibrations that some of us spoke of some years ago. We have to have the fantasy first, and then we try to put it into action.

Michael Conran (U.K.). I very much enjoyed Dr. Meissner's presentation, and I have asked myself what exactly was the quality in it that appealed to me. I think I discovered it in his subsequent remarks. It is his love of precision. I personally have great difficulty in being precise, so I am going to try very hard to be precise about my imprecision. I belong to the body of so-called independent psychoanalysts in London, and without being a declared Kleinian, I cannot imagine myself working without the concept of projective identification. To me it represents not only a splitting mechanism in the mind, and the projection of a part of the self, with attendant unwanted feelings linked to another person or persons, but also something which is inevitably accompanied by regression and dependency. This is because one part of the self has been split off. This is generally the adult part of the self, the governing part, the understanding, the part of the self that is going to experience pain and has to suffer that pain. Once that has happened, the individual has to some extent infantilized himself, made himself childlike, but that is not all. Once that part of the self is lodged in somebody else it must be attended to in that other person, so the individual becomes dependent on the other. There is to my mind no question but that projective identification is accompanied by the two defensive measures of regression and dependency.

We come now to the area that Dr. Meissner does not like, which he finds imprecise. Anyone who has worked with schizophrenics in a mental hospital will have seen how they split off and push bits of themselves into a variety of different people in the institution. Then, of course, they have to spend their lives going around from one to another, attending to these different bits of themselves. If we move from the mental hospital to a court of law, we may see a derelict, empty, silent individual in the dock, a person in whom all the feelings and all the argument, all the living parts are contained in a variety of different people—the judge, the prosecuting counsel, the police, the witnesses, the defending counsel, and so forth. Those who have experienced severe illness will know how unable they were to govern themselves while they were totally preoccupied with their internal feelings and their wish to escape, somehow or other, from something they could neither understand nor manage, from unmanageable anxiety. Such individuals then place themselves in the hands of their doctor or their surgeon. In these circumstances the governing of themselves is split off entirely and pushed into other people, and then, as this matter is dealt with, they are able to take back these projected bits of themselves and cease to be helpless babies. We used to say, of male patients in hospitals, that when the fellow gets better and takes an interest in the nurses' ankles, it is time to discharge him.

In analysis one sees this in many different ways. I will simply give one instance, which must accord with the experience of many people, and that is of the patient who has no associations. The analyst finds himself having the patient's associations. How does this come about? This raises, of course, the whole question of the nature of the countertransference experience. Now all I want to say about Dr. Meissner's clinical examples is to ask him what he felt when the patient came into the room and told him about what he wanted to do with the machine gun. What would Dr. Meissner's feelings be in relation to making a transference interpretation about that? What did he think the patient might do?

W. W. Meissner. There is so much that is rich and challenging in the comments that I may do a disservice to many of you who contributed, and for this I give my apologies in advance. Perhaps a first blanket comment might be in order. Certainly, in response to what Dr. Sandler said, one of the methodological difficulties we continue to face is the interplay between clinical experience and our attempt to think about that experience. Whatever one's theoretical orientation, it is clear that the material that patients provide us is full of content. It is riddled with fantasies of all kinds, and that serves as a basis for what we try to process and understand about what goes on inside the minds of our patients. The radical dichotomies that have so often been proposed that would pose fantasy and content against theory, process, and mechanism are very artificial, and I am sure that when analysts reach the point where they are actually talking about what is happening with the patient, they have a common ground. That is very important for us to keep in mind.

If we look at the issue of the delicate interplay that takes place within the transference, many of my remarks were focused on transference, but not particularly focused on countertransference. In this I defer to Dr. Kernberg, because clearly that is his contribution to our work in this conference. But obviously everyone is attuned to and understands the fact that when these processes come into play in the analytic relationship, the analyst reacts, things are being elicited from him, the analyst has sensitivities and finds himself drawn into particular positions. For example, during the break, someone asked me about my second case, and said, "My goodness, how difficult it must have been to stand by and to watch this lady on her self-defeating course, where she was getting herself divorced, and not doing anything to protect her interests." Quite obviously this was a very difficult situation for the analyst. The patient adopted a position of passivity and victimization, and the analyst was invited to take a more aggressive stance, to join the dance with her, if you will, around this issue. To what extent does one do that? How much does one take the initiative to try to impress upon her, let us say, the difficulty that she is getting into? How much does one take the role of the aggressor that she herself should be taking? How much does one avoid the countertransference trap, and to what extent does it facilitate the work of the analyst to do one or the other? The important thing here is that one should be aware of these things taking place, just as with my first case, in which the man had near-psychotic delusions of shooting up the place, and so on. Well, I felt very threatened. There was no question but that he was generating a context within the transference where my countertransference response was to feel myself in a position of vulnerability, and in the role of victim.

What does one say about the kinds of experience I have just referred to? Is it necessarily the case that we are witnessing projective identification? What we witness can be put in very different terms, and can be seen as an interplay between a projective process on one side and an introjective process on the other, further compounded by the generation of a counterprojective process that can induce another layer of introjection in the patient, within this complex interaction. Are we forced to think that projective identification is involved in any situation of interaction in which something is elicited collusively from an object, an eliciting that may have been determined to some extent by a projection from the subject? I am not persuaded that that is at all necessary, and again my concern is the implication of the terminology as we use it. Is it an identification? I think everyone would agree that there is projection involved in this complex interaction, but is an identification involved? Again, what does one mean by an identification? My use of identification tends to be much more specific, tends to run to a much more integrated, more secondary process kind of phenomenon, to internalizations that have a positive, constructive autonomy-building effect. When one uses the term projective identification, that is not *my* identification. That is a much more primitive kind of process that has to do with defensive needs, the determination of drive elements, and a whole host of things that speak to me of a process taking place on a less autonomous, often defensively derived basis. So there are many complex issues here that one needs to think about. If one is in the habit of thinking about this kind of complex phenomenon as connected with a particular terminology, then it becomes very difficult to pull back from that and to say what the implications are of the terminology. I find myself hesitant about that kind of approach, and relatively unsympathetic toward it.

I want to make one focused remark that might otherwise get lost in the discussion. I am sure that Dr. Kernberg is aware that a very radical selection of elements from Klein and Bion had to be made, with a certain focus in mind, and I am sure that the selection I made could have been better and perhaps different. If I were doing it again I might make a different selection, but the methodological point that Dr. Kernberg raised is, I think, a very important one. The issue involved is that of how one understands the process of internalization. To put it very succinctly, my notion of internalization is that what is brought inside becomes a part of the internal organization of the personality, of the psychic structure. It is integrated into the organization of the self. Now the whole issue of whether internalizations take place only in terms of self-representations hinges on the point of whether the internalization is brought into the compass of the object relationship. But we are still talking of the inner world. We are talking of the representational world. We are talking about something that is not synonymous with psychic structure or with the internal integration of the self-organization. I think one has to keep many layers and complexities of distinction in mind in order to begin to sort out the complexities involved. I am sure we will have ample opportunity to explore these further, but I am pleased and delighted that these issues have surfaced so early in our discussion.

Chapter 5

Projective Identification: Clinical Aspects

BETTY JOSEPH

The concept of projective identification was introduced into analytic thinking by Melanie Klein in 1946. Since then it has been welcomed, argued about, the name disputed, the links with projection pointed out, and so on; but one aspect seems to stand out above the firing line, and that is its considerable clinical value. It is this aspect that I shall concentrate on today, mainly in relation to the more neurotic patient.

Melanie Klein became aware of projective identification when exploring what she called the paranoid-schizoid position, that is, a constellation of a particular type of object relations, anxieties, and defenses against them, typical for the earliest period of the individual's life and, in certain disturbed people, continuing throughout life. This particular position she saw as dominated by the infant's need to ward off anxieties and impulses by splitting both the object, originally the mother, and the self and projecting these split-off parts into an object, which will then be felt to be like, or identified with, these split-off parts, so coloring the infant's perception of the object and its subsequent introjection.

She discussed the manifold aims of different types of projective identification, for example, splitting off and getting rid of unwanted parts of the self that cause anxiety or pain; projecting the self or parts of the self into an object to dominate and control it and thus avoid any feelings of being separate; getting into an object to take over its capacities and make them its own; invading in order to damage or destroy the object. Thus the infant, or adult who goes on using such mechanisms powerfully, can avoid any awareness of separateness, dependence, or admiration or of the

65

concomitant sense of loss, anger, envy, etc. But it sets up persecutory anxieties, claustrophobia, panics, and the like.

We could say that, from the point of view of the individual who uses such mechanisms strongly, projective identification is a fantasy, and yet it can have a powerful effect on the recipient. It does not always do so and when it does we cannot always tell how the effect is brought about, but we cannot doubt its importance. We can see, however, that the concept of projective identification, used in this way, is more object-related and more concrete, and covers more aspects than the term projection would ordinarily imply, and it has opened up a whole area of analytic understanding. These various aspects I am going to discuss later, as we see them operating in our clinical work; here I want only to stress two points: first, the omnipotent power of these mechanisms and fantasies; second, how insofar as they originate in a particular constellation, deeply interlocked, we cannot in our thinking isolate projective identification from the omnipotence, the splitting, and the anxieties that attend it. Indeed, we shall see that they are all part of a balance, rigidly or precariously maintained by the individual, in his own unique way.

As the individual develops, either in normal development or through analytic treatment, these projections lessen, he becomes more able to tolerate his ambivalence, his love and hate and dependence on objects. In other words, he moves toward what Melanie Klein described as the depressive position. This process can be helped in infancy if the child has a supportive environment, if the mother is able to tolerate and contain the child's projections, intuitively to understand and stand its feelings. Bion elaborated and extended this aspect of Melanie Klein's work, suggesting the importance of the mother's being able to be used as a container by the infant, and linking this with the process of communication in childhood and with the positive use of the countertransference in analysis. Once the child is better integrated and able to recognize its impulses and feelings as its own, there will be a lessening in the pressure to project, accompanied by an increased concern for the object. In its earliest forms projective identification has no concern for the object; indeed, often it is an anticoncern aimed at dominating, irrespective of the cost to the object. As the child moves toward the depressive position this necessarily alters; although projective identification is probably never entirely given up, it will no longer involve the complete splitting off and disowning of parts of the self, but will be less absolute, more temporary, and more able to be drawn back into the individual's personality—and thus be the basis of empathy.

In this paper I want first to consider some further implications of the use of projective identification, and then to discuss and illustrate various aspects of it, first in two patients more or less stuck in the paranoid-schizoid position, and then in one beginning to move toward the depressive position.

To begin with, some of the implications, clinical and technical, of the massive use of projective identification as we see it in our work: Sometimes it is used so massively that we get the impression that the patient is in fantasy projecting his whole self into his object and may feel trapped or claustrophobic. It is, in any case, a very powerful and effective way of ridding the individual of contact with his own mind; at times the mind can be so weakened or so fragmented by splitting processes, or so evacuated by projective identification, that the individual appears empty or quasi-psychotic. This I shall show in the case of C, a child. Projective identification also has important technical implications; for example, the fact that it is but one aspect of an omnipotent balance established by each individual in his own way any interpretive attempt on the part of the analyst to locate and give back to the patient missing parts of the self must of necessity be resisted by the total personality, since it is felt to threaten the whole balance and lead to more disturbance. This I shall discuss in the case of T. Projective identification cannot be seen in isolation.

A further clinical implication that I should like to touch on involves communication. Bion demonstrated how projective identification can be used as a method of communication by the individual, who, as it were, puts undigested parts of his experience and inner world into the object, originally the mother, and now the analyst, as a way of getting them understood and returned in a more manageable form. But we might add to this that projective identification is by its very nature a kind of communication, even in cases where this is not its aim. By definition projective identification means the putting of parts of the self into an object. If the analyst on the receiving end is really open to what is going on and able to be aware of what he is experiencing, this can be a powerful method of gaining understanding. Indeed, much of our current appreciation of the richness of the notion of countertransference stems from it. I shall later try to indicate some of the problems this raises, in terms of acting in, in my discussion of the third case, that of N.

I want now to illustrate, with the case of C, the concreteness of projective identification in the analytic situation, its effectiveness as a method of ridding the child of a whole area of experience and thus keeping some kind of balance, and the effect of such massive projective mechanisms on her state of mind. This is a little girl of four, in analytic treatment with Mrs. Rocha Barros, who was discussing the case with me. The child, neglected and deeply disturbed, had only very recently begun treatment.

A few minutes before the end of a Friday session C said that she was going to make a candle; the analyst explained her wish to take a warm Mrs. Barros with her that day at the end of the session and her fear that there would not be enough time, as there were only three minutes left. C started to scream, saying that she would have some spare candles; she then started to stare through the window with a vacant, lost expression. The analyst interpreted that the child needed to make the analyst realize how awful it was to end the session, as well as expressing a wish to take home some warmth from the analyst's words for the weekend. The child screamed: "Bastard! Take off your clothes and jump outside." Again the analyst tried to interpret C's feelings about being dropped and sent into the cold. C replied: "Stop your talking, take off your clothes. You are cold. I'm not cold." The feeling in the session was extremely moving. Here the words carry the concrete meaning, to the child, of the separation of the weekend—the awful coldness. This she tries to force into the analyst, and it is felt to have been concretely achieved. "You are cold; I am not cold."

The moments when C looked completely lost and vacant, as in this fragment, were very frequent and were, I think, indicative not only of her serious loss of contact with reality, but of the emptiness, the vacantness of her mind and personality when projective identification was operating so powerfully. I think that much of her screaming is also in the nature of this emptying out. The effectiveness of such emptying is striking, as the whole experience of loss and its concomitant emotions is cut out. One can see here how the term projective identification describes more vividly and fully the processes involved than the more general and frequently used terms, such as "reversal" or "projection."

In this example, then, the child's balance is primarily maintained by the projecting out of parts of the self. I want now to give an example of a familiar kind of case to illustrate various kinds of projective identification working together to hold a particular narcissistic omnipotent balance. This kind of balance is very firmly structured, is extremely difficult to influence analytically, and leads to striking persecutory anxieties. It also raises some points about different identificatory processes and about problems with the term projective identification.

A young teacher, whom I shall call T, came into analysis with difficulties in relationships, but actually with the hope of changing careers and becoming an analyst. His daily material consisted very largely of descriptions of work he had done in helping his pupils, how his colleagues had praised his work, asked him to discuss their work with him, and so on. Little else came into the sessions. He frequently described how one or another of his colleagues felt threatened by him, threatened in the sense of feeling minimized or put in an inferior position by his greater insight and understanding. He was therefore uneasy that they might feel unfriendly toward him. (Any idea that his personality might actually put people off did not enter his mind.) It was not difficult to show him that he held similar ideas about me—for example, that I did not encourage him to give up his career and apply for training as an analyst, because, being old, I felt threatened by this intelligent young person.

Clearly, to interpret that T was projecting his envy into his objects and then feeling them as identified with this part of himself would be clinically inept and useless, however theoretically accurate, as it would just be absorbed into his psychoanalytic armory. We can see that the projective identification of the envious parts of the self was only the end result of one aspect of a highly complex balance he was maintaining. To clarify the nature of this balance, it is important to see how T was relating to me in the transference. Usually he spoke of me as a very fine analyst and I was flattered in such ways. Actually he could not take in interpretations meaningfully, and appeared not to listen properly; for example, he would hear my words only partially, reinterpret them unconsciously according to some theoretical psychoanalytic understanding he had, and then give them to himself with this slightly altered and generalized meaning. Frequently, when I interpreted more firmly, he would respond very quickly and argumentatively, as if a minor explosion were set off that not only would expel from his mind what I might be going to say, but would enter my mind and break up my thinking at that moment.

In this example we have projective identification operating with various motives and leading to different identificatory processes—all aimed at maintaining a narcissistic omnipotent balance. First we see the splitting of his objects—I am flattered and kept in his mind as idealized while my bad or unhelpful aspect is quite split off. Though I don't seem to be achieving much with him, this must be denied. He projects part of himself into my mind and takes over; he "knows" what I am going to say and says it himself. At this point, a part of the self is identified with an idealized aspect of myself, which is talking to, interpreting to, an idealized patient part of himself—idealized because it listens to the analyst part of him. We can see what this movement achieves in terms of his balance. It cuts out any real relationship between the patient and myself, between patient and analyst, as a feeding couple, as mother and child. It obviates any separate existence, any relating to me as myself—any relationship in which he takes in directly from me. T was, in fact, earlier in his life slightly anorexic. If I manage for a moment to get through this, T explodes; his mental digestive system is thereby fragmented, and by this verbal explosion, as I have noted, T unconsciously tries to enter my mind and break up my thinking, my capacity to feed him. It is important here, as always with projective identification, to distinguish this kind of unconscious entering, invading, and breaking up from a conscious aggressive attack. What I am discussing here is how these patients, using projective identification so omnipotently, actually avoid such feelings as dependence, envy, jealousy, etc.

Once T has in fantasy entered my mind and taken over my interpretations, and my role at that moment, I notice that he has "added to," "improved on," "enriched" my interpretations, and I become the onlooker, who should realize that my interpretations of a few moments ago were not as rich as his are now—and surely I should feel threatened by this young man in my room! Thus the two types of projective identification are working in harmony, the invading of my mind and taking over its contents and the projecting of the potentially dependent, threatened, and envious part of the self into me. This is, of course, mirrored in what we hear is going on in his outside world—the fellow teachers who ask for help and feel threatened by his brilliance—but then he feels persecuted by their potential unfriendliness. So long as the balance holds so effectively, we cannot see that more subtle, sensitive, and important aspects of the personality are being kept split off, or why—we can see only that any relationship to a truly separate object is obviated, with all that this may imply.

A great difficulty, of course, is that all insight tends to get drawn into this process. To give an example, one Monday T seemed to become aware of exactly how he was subtly taking the meaning out of what I was saying and not letting real understanding develop. For a moment he felt relief, and then a brief, deep feeling of hatred of me emerged into consciousness. A second later he added quietly that he was thinking how the way that he had been feeling just then toward me, that is, the hatred, must have been how his fellow students had felt toward him the previous day, when he had been talking and explaining things to them! So no sooner has T a real experience of hating me, because I have said something useful, than he uses this momentary awareness to speak about the students, thus distancing himself from the emerging envy and hostility and losing the direct receptive contact between us. What looks like insight is no longer insight but has become a complex projective maneuver.

At a period when these problems were very much in the forefront of the analysis, T brought up a dream, right at the end of a session. The dream was simply this: T was with the analyst or with a woman, J, or it might have been both. He was excitedly pushing his hand up her knickers into her vagina, thinking that if he could get right in there would be no stopping him. Here, I think under the pressure of the analytic work going on, T's great need and great excitement was to get totally inside the object, with all its implications, including, of course, the annihilation of the analytic situation.

To return to the concept of projective identification, with this patient I have indicated three or four different aspects: attacking the analyst's mind; a kind of total invading, as in the dream fragment above; a more partial invasion and takeover of aspects or capacities of the analyst; and, finally, putting parts of the self, particularly inferior parts, into the analyst. The latter two aspects are mutually dependent, but lead to different types of identification. In the one, the patient, in taking over, becomes identified with the analyst's idealized capacities; in the other, it is the analyst who becomes identified with the lost, projected, here inferior or envious parts of the patient. I think it is partly because the term is broad and covers these many aspects that there has been some uneasiness regarding it.

I have so far discussed projective identification in two cases caught up in the paranoid-schizoid position, a borderline child and a man in a rigid omnipotent narcissistic state. Now I want to discuss aspects of projective identification as seen in a patient moving toward the depressive position. I shall present material from the case of a man as he was becoming less rigid, more integrated, better able to tolerate what was previously projected, but constantly also pulling back, returning to the use of the earlier projective mechanisms; then I want to show the effect of this on subsequent identifications and the light that it throws on previous ones. I want also to forge a link between the nature of the patient's residual use of projective identification and its early infantile counterpart, and to show how this relates to phobia formation. I will also discuss briefly the communicative nature of projective identification.

To start with this last point, as projective identification is by its very nature the putting of parts of the self into the object, in the transference we are of necessity on the receiving end of the projections; therefore, providing we can tune into them, we have an opportunity par excellence to understand what is going on. In this sense, projective identification acts as a communication, whatever its motivation, and is the basis for the positive use of countertransference. As with this patient, N, it is frequently difficult to determine whether, at any given moment, projective identification is aimed primarily at communicating a state of mind that cannot be verbalized by the patient or whether it is aimed more at entering and controlling (or attacking) the analyst. Often both aims are present and require consideration.

A patient, N, who had been in analysis many years, had recently married. After a few weeks, he was becoming anxious about his sexual interest and his potency, particularly in view of the fact that his wife was considerably younger. He came in on a Monday saying he felt that "the thing" was never really going to get right, "the sexual thing." Yes, they did have sex on Sunday, but somehow he had to force himself; he knew it wasn't quite right, and his wife noticed this and commented. It was an all right kind of weekend, just about. He spoke about this a bit more and explained that they had gone to a place outside London, to a party. They had meant to stay the night in a hotel nearby, but couldn't find a place nice enough and so came home very late. What was being conveyed to me was a quiet, sad discomfort, leading to despair, and I pointed out to N how he was conveying an awful, long-term hopelessness and despair, with no hope for the future. He replied to the effect that he supposed that he was feeling left out, and linked this with what had been a rather helpful and vivid session that Friday; but now, as he made the remark, the session seemed dead and flat. When I tried to look at this with him, he agreed, commenting that he supposed he was starting to attack the analysis. The feeling in the session now was awful; N was making a kind of sense and saying analytic things which could have been right, for example about the Friday, and which one could have picked up; but, since they seemed flat and quite unhelpful to him, what he seemed to me to be doing was putting despair into me, not only about the reality of his marriage and his potency, but also about his analysis. This was indicated, for example, by the useless and by now somewhat irrelevant comment about being left out. N denied my interpretation about his despair over the progress of the analysis, but in such a way, it seemed to me, as to be encouraging me to make false interpretations and to pick up his pseudointerpretations as if I believed in them, while knowing full well that they and we were getting nowhere. He spoke vaguely about this but then went quiet and said: "I was listening to your voice, the timbre changes in different voices. W [his wife], being younger, makes more sounds per second; older voices are deeper because they make less sounds per second, etc." With my voice, rather than through my actual words, I showed N his great fear that I could not stand the extent of his hopelessness and his doubts about myself, about what we could achieve in the analysis and in his life, and that I would cheat and in some way try to encourage him. I asked whether he had perhaps felt that in that session my voice had changed in order to sound more encouraging and encouraged, rather than contain the despair he was expressing. By this point in the session my patient had got back into contact and said, with some relief, that if I did do this kind of encouraging the whole bottom would fall out of the analysis.

First, the nature of the communication, which I was able to understand primarily through my countertransference, through the way in which I was being pushed and pulled to feel and to react: We see here the concrete quality of projective identification structuring the countertransference. N was not asking me to understand the sexual difficulties or the unhappiness, but rather was invading me with despair, while at the same time unconsciously trying to force me to reassure myself that it was all right, that interpretations, now empty of meaning and hollow, were meaningful, and that the analysis at that moment was proceeding satisfactorily. Thus it was not only the despair that N was projecting into me, but his defenses against it, a false reassurance and denial he intended I should act out with him. I think that this also suggests a projective identification of an internal figure, primarily his mother, who was felt to be weak, kind, but unable to stand up to emotion. In the transference (to oversimplify the picture) this figure was projected into me, and I found myself pushed to live it out.

We have here the important issue of teasing out the motivation for this projective identification: was it aimed primarily at communicating something to me? Was there a depth of despair that previously we had not sufficiently understood? Or was this forcing of despair into me motivated by something different? At this stage, at the end of the session, I did not know and so left it open.

I have so much condensed the material here that I cannot convey adequately the atmosphere and the to-and-fro of the session. But toward the end, as I have tried to show, my patient experienced and expressed relief and appreciation of what had been going on. There was a shift in mood and behavior as my patient started to accept understanding and to face the nature of his forcing his mental contents into me, and he could then experience me as an object that could stand up to his acting in, not get caught up in it, but contain it. He could then identify temporarily with a stronger object, and he himself became firmer. I also sensed some feeling of concern about what he had been doing to me and to my work; this was not openly acknowledged and expressed, but there was some movement toward the depressive position, with its real concern and guilt.

To clarify the motivation as well as the effect of this kind of projective identification on subsequent introjective identification, we need to go briefly into the beginning of the next session, when N brought in a dream. He was on a boat like a ferry boat, on a grey-green sea surrounded by mist; he did not know where they were going. Then nearby there was another boat which was clearly going down under the water and drowning. He stepped onto this boat as it went down. He did not feel wet or afraid, which was puzzling. Among his associations we heard of his wife being very gentle and affectionate, but he added that he himself was concerned that behind this she might really be making more demands on him. She, knowing his fondness for steak and kidney pudding, had made him one the night before. It was excellent, but the taste was too strong, which he told her!

Now the interesting thing, I think, was that on the previous day I had felt rather at sea, not knowing exactly where we were going, but was clear that my understanding about the hopelessness and his defenses against it was right; though I had not thought it out in this way, my belief would have been that the mists would clear as we went on. But what does my patient do with this? He gratuitously steps off this boat (this understanding) onto one that is going down, and he is not afraid! In other words, he prefers to drown in despair rather than clarify it, prefers to see affection as demands, and views my decent, well-cooked steak and kidney interpretations as too tasty. At this point, as we worked on it, N could see that the notion of drowning here was actually exciting to him.

Now we can see more about the motivation. It becomes clear that N was not just trying to communicate and get understood something about his despair, important as this element is, but that he was also attacking me and our work, by trying to drag me down by the despair, when in fact progress was being made. After a session in which he expressed appreciation for my work and my capacity to stand up to him, he dreamt of willingly stepping onto a sinking boat; internally, I must either collide and go down with him or watch him go under, my hope destroyed and impotent to help. This activity also leads to an introjective identification with an analyst-parent who is felt to be down, joyless, and impotent, and this identification contributes considerably to his lack of sexual confidence and potency. Following this period of the analysis, there was real improvement in the symptom.

Naturally these considerations lead one to think about the nature of the patient's internal objects (for example, the weak mother) that I described as being projected into me in the transference. How much is this figure based on N's real experience with his mother, and how much did he exploit her weaknesses and thus contribute to building in his inner world a mother weak, inadequate, and on the defensive, as we saw in the transference? In other words, when we talk of an object projected onto the analyst in the transference, we are discussing an internal object that has been structured in part from the child's earlier projective identifications, and the whole process can be seen being revived in the transference.

I want now to digress and look at this material from a slightly different angle, related to the patient's very early history and anxieties. I have shown how N pulls back and goes into an object—in the dream, into the sinking boat—as in the first session he goes into despair, which he then projects into me rather than having to think about it. This going into an object, acted out in the session, is, I believe, linked with a type of projective identification more total than that indicated in the sexual dream of T or seen in connection with phobia formation. At the very primitive end of projective identification is the attempt to get back into an object, to become, as it were, undifferentiated and mindless, thus avoiding all pain. Although most human beings develop beyond this in early infancy, some of our patients attempt to use projective identification in this way over many years. N came into analysis because he had a fetish, a tremendous pull toward getting inside a rubber object which would totally cover, absorb, and excite him. In his early childhood he had had nightmares of falling out of a globe into endless space. In the early period of analysis he would have severe panic states when alone in the house, and would be seriously disturbed or lose contact if he had to be out of town on business. At the same time there were minor indications of anxieties about claustrophobic entrapment. For example, at night he would have to keep the bedclothes loose or throw them off altogether; in intercourse, fantasies emerged of his penis being cut off and lost inside the woman's body. As the analysis went on, the fetishistic activities disappeared, real relationships improved, and the projecting of self into object could clearly be seen in the transference. He would become absorbed in the sound of his own words, or of mine, the meaning of which would be unimportant compared with the concrete nature of the experience. This absorption into words and sounds with the analyst, quite disregarded as a person, is not unlike a process sometimes seen in child patients: they come into the playroom, climb onto the couch, and fall so deeply asleep that interpretations do not wake them. It is interesting to see how N has always attempted to get concretely into an object, apparently to escape being outside, to become absorbed and free of relating, of thought and mental pain. And yet we know this is only half the story, as the principal object he entered was a highly sexualized fetish. And still, in the dream of getting into the sinking boat, there was masochistic excitement that he tried to pull me into; in this sense the dream may be compared to that of T. Earlier as T's constant invading and taking over was being analyzed, I described how we could see in his sexual dream an attempt to get totally inside of me, with great excitement. I suspect there is much yet to be teased out about the relation between erotization and certain types of massive projective identification of the self.

I want now to consider the question of projective identification in patients who, becoming more integrated, are approaching the depressive position. We can see that with N—unlike T, who is still imprisoned in his own omnipotent narcissistic structure—there is now a movement in the transference toward more genuine, whole object relations. At times he can really appreciate the strong containing qualities of his object; true, he may then try to draw me in and drag me down again, but there is now a potential for conflict over this. The object can be valued and loved—at times he can consciously experience hostility about this—and ambivalence is present. As his loving is freed he is able to introject and identify with a whole object, valued and potent, and the effect on his character and potency is striking. This kind of identification is very different from the process of forcing despairing parts of the self into an object who then in fantasy becomes a despairing part of the self. It is very different from the identification we saw in T, whereby the patient invaded my mind and took over the split-off idealized aspects, leaving the object denuded and inferior. By contrast, N could experience and value me as a whole and properly separate person with my own qualities, and these he could introject thereby feeling strengthened. But ahead lies the task of enabling N to be truly outside—to give up the analysis, aware of its meaning to him and yet secure.

Chapter 6

Discussion of Betty Joseph's Paper

Joseph Sandler.   Betty Joseph has shown us that in her work there is certainly an appropriate place for the concept of projective identification. She has also shown us that it can have different meanings, that it is not one thing, but rather a constellation of processes in which we see different aspects at different times.

This paper has presented us some very interesting clinical material, and its relevance for us is for our understanding of processes of internalization and externalization, projective identification in particular. I think we are all aware that projective identification is a concept that has had different meanings for different people, or even different meanings for the same person at different times. So we have to ask ourselves where we stand in relation to the different usages to be found in Betty Joseph's paper. In England just after the Second World War, a law was enacted to prevent shopkeepers from refusing to sell a scarce article unless the purchaser bought something else along with it. It became illegal to make a package deal, as it was called. I will not say it is illegal to buy Betty Joseph's whole package, and everyone is free to do so; but everyone also has the right to concentrate on projective identification only, without having to buy the other aspects of the paper as well. I say this to make it clear that although the concept was introduced by Melanie Klein, one does not, by accepting it and finding it useful, automatically become a Kleinian. This is important, because there are many of us who are not Kleinians and yet have found the notion to be important.

I was very struck how much the paper reflects a shift in psychoanalytic thinking away from the idea that behavior is more or less directly a drive derivative. Throughout the paper there is the notion of maintaining a balance, of using defenses to restore narcissistic equilibrium. This is very important; as Betty Joseph has pointed out, projective identification is object-related, and we involve our objects in maintaining our inner equilibrium. We all live in an object world that is not only external but internal, and we have to maintain a balance throughout development in relation to both internal and external objects. Defensive processes are very important in maintaining that balance. It is natural then that the patient might have a resistance to direct interpretation of a mechanism he is using to restore his balance, or to maintain it; if he were to accept the interpretation, his balance would be upset. In the fantasy life of the individual, defensive fantasies involving interactions between self and object are created from past and present material in order to maintain balance. In this we have to take account not only of drives but also of a secondary motivating system; this is perhaps not a phrase that Betty Joseph would use, but I hope that my meaning will be clear. Throughout the descriptions we have been given are references to ways of dealing with envy, rage, anxiety, hopelessness, and other feelings. All these disturb the balance and have to be controlled, and I was very happy to see this notion implicit in the paper. I hope that it will become more explicit, because I am convinced that with the increasing emphasis on the relationships to external and internal objects, analysis will have to adopt a double theory of motivation. I refer here to drives on the one hand, and, on the other, all those other motives essentially linked with painful feelings. Well, those are my own immediate thoughts, and I will confine myself to them at present.

   Lars Sjögren (Sweden).   I have been working with the concept of projective identification for a long time, but it has not transformed me into a Kleinian. The package we were presented evoked a lot of thoughts in me, and I have selected two of these to speak about. The first is the fact that projective identification is a communication, a bridge, and to build a bridge one needs two bridgeheads. We have done very little research on the bridgehead from the side of the analyst. We are very interested in what the analysand communicates through projective identification, but we should ask how this communication enters the analyst. What is there in the analyst that makes this possible? Of course this is what we sometimes call countertransference, but countertransference is often a word that allows one to escape the awareness of some attitude that arises in and belongs to the analyst, and which is evoked by a particular patient. The patient may have unconsciously become aware of this attitude, and built his communication to the analyst on something that he or she unconsciously knows about. So to what extent should we admit, in the first case mentioned by Miss Joseph, that the analyst was cold in the way she was going to leave the patient over the weekend? It has become standard to say, "You have this dream because it is just before the weekend," or, "It is because I am going to leave you for a conference in Jerusalem." We do this regularly, but there are other things we do, things we don't wish to dwell on. In your last case, for example, you were older than he is, and at a certain moment he was cleverer than you because he made you confused. To what extent should you talk about that? Of course there is no general answer to this, but there might be something to talk about with the patient. How far should we go without losing our analytic stance and still avoid pushing pathology which does not belong there into the patient? The crucial point is, I think, whether to admit something that exists in reality. It is what we do when we open the door to the patient a minute too late, and the patient reacts in some way, and we say, "This is your answer to the fact that I opened the door a minute too late." I think we have here a field of research for analysts.

I was very interested in your last case, Miss Joseph. He was not psychotic, but you could point out the projective identification occurring. This is important for all of us who want to see the process going on, but I should like to ask whether it is a healthy thing for the patient to allow the sequence to occur. I am talking about benevolent patients who are not using projective identification in order to destroy the analyst. Would it not be healthier if first the analyst became confused and then came back with a good interpretation? I mean healthy in the sense that this prevents an omnipotent projective identification from the patient into the analyst. If the analyst can show the analysand that the analyst is not really omnipotent, that she is confused and doesn't understand the patient, but comes back the next day and does understand, then this is on a more human level than if the patient had been understood immediately. It would have then been easier for the patient to keep the analyst in an omnipotent position and more difficult for him to do the "healthy" work of introjecting you as a separate person with your own qualities. And among your own qualities is the capacity to become confused and in some way to admit it and still help the patient. This is something I have been wondering about in my own work, because I have the impression that patients do gain a lot from periods of confusion on my part.

Joseph Sandler. I think you have made your point very clearly. What you stress, of course, is the technical problem of interpreting the counter-transference and telling the patient about reality, and thus not pretending to be omnipotent.

Betty Joseph. I do think that these points are of great importance when we look at the technical problem of handling projective identifications. As you know, some people, including Mrs. Klein, really prefer to keep the word countertransference mainly or entirely for the analyst's unhealthy response. The analyst has to take it back to his or her own analyst, if there is one. In my paper I preferred to see the idea of projective identification in terms of what the patient made the analyst feel.

Coming now to the bridgeheads, it seems to me that we ought, as people who have been analyzed, to be reasonably clear about how much of what is aroused in us comes primarily from our own pathology and shouldn't be acted out with the patient. It belongs somewhere else. Let us take my case of the teacher. He was certainly much better read analytically than I am, and when he came into analysis he at first read more or less nothing but works on psychoanalysis. Of course I pointed out to him that he was perfectly aware of my age, of my growing-older quality. However, what I pointed out to him as well is how he responds to it, and how he assumes that I feel left out, that I feel rather tragic about it and envious. Now if I really did feel envious of this man I would need to consider that as my own problem, but I am afraid he doesn't really inspire much envy. But suppose he did; I should still be able to distinguish that from what my patient wishes to stir up in me. To my mind this is an extremely important distinction. I certainly feel that it is not appropriate to do what is called "admitting our feelings"; they belong to us and to our analysis. We need to distinguish very carefully what our patient unconsciously wishes us to feel, and how he reacts to such facts as age or being Jewish or this or that which cannot be denied. These things are facts which we must take as background, but we must not work out our problems with our patients nor burden them with our feelings. If, for example, a patient thinks that I have responded too hastily and therefore takes it that I was angry with him, then I would say, "I think you felt I responded too hastily, and then you felt that this must mean I felt this and this," leaving out entirely what I actually felt.

I was asked whether it might be healthier for the patient if the analyst allowed the sequence to occur of helplessness, followed by interpretation the following day. Otherwise, if I understand the questioner correctly, one might reply too quickly, interpret too quickly, and then appear omnipotent. I think this was the point of the question. I want to say that there is not a chance that I would omnipotently be so quick because with this man, as with all these patients, it takes a long time within a session to feel what the patient is expressing, to be aware, from the "drag" of the session, of something of, say, the patient's hopelessness and despair. So it is going to take a long time before I can understand this, and therefore I can only build up very slowly the picture for my patient of what I think he is trying to convey. There is very little risk if one works this way of being too quick or too clever, and therefore appearing to one's patient to be omnipotent. If this happens, then one has to sort out with one's patient how he feels that one was being too quick or omnipotent, and to point out his anger about that.

Joseph Sandler. This is a very important technical point, and I am glad it was raised. Perhaps I might take the liberty of making one small comment. Sometimes when patients externalize in the way Betty Joseph has described, they do so knowing unconsciously very well which buttons to press in the analyst in order to get a particular response, and they are capable of making one feel envious, for example. One feels as if this is one's own problem (and it often is), but it has been prompted, stimulated, evoked by the patient. It becomes extraordinarily difficult to differentiate this from what is described as straightforward projective identification. Sometimes one cannot really differentiate the two until some sort of crisis has been reached in the countertransference. A point comes where one has to sit down and think very hard about what is going on, or even take advice. I am not sure that the clear differentiation which Betty Joseph makes is so clear in practice.

Otto Kernberg. This was a paper of an extraordinary level of sophistication and clinical work, and we don't often have the opportunity to hear a presentation of this sort. I should like to add something to the discussion on countertransference. While I very much agree with what Betty Joseph proposed in regard to the concept and to the technical handling of the patient, with very sick—borderline or psychotic—patients there may be onslaughts of acting out in the transference that are so intense that to contain them makes the analyst experience a regression in his countertransference. This complements projective identification, so that the fact that the analyst sees that he is reacting with countertransference responses that are very personal does not necessarily mean that he is experiencing countertransference in the restricted way which Betty Joseph mentioned. While one should separate what comes from oneself from that which comes from the patient, with very sick patients we get something like a compromise formation that includes elements both from the patient and from one's own self. But that should not preclude analyzing this in the course of one's work with the patient. If it is too intense, as Dr. Sandler has indicated, then one works on it outside the sessions. With very sick patients I find myself often working things through between the sessions, and I don't consider that it indicates that there is anything wrong with me. Again, in regard to countertransference, Miss Joseph mentioned that projective identification initiates counter-transference, and I would say that it particularly originates a type of countertransference, that which Racker called complementary identifica-tion in the countertransference. Other processes permit more concordant types of identification, in which the analyst identifies with the central subjective experience of the patient. It is an introjective type of identifica-tion which generates countertransference reactions of a different kind. It seems to me that there are oscillations between concordant and comple-mentary types of identification and countertransference which are de-pendent on whether the analyst identifies either with the patient's self or with the patient's projected objects. Of course, sometimes the patient identifies with his own object and the analyst identifies with the patient's self. In this connection, the patient T became like his students, relating to you, who were him; and although you didn't say how you handled that, one could interpret it by saying, "You are now talking about the student because you are trying to avoid your feeling like a student to me." This illustrates the diadic self and object component activated during projec-tive identification.

What I particularly enjoyed in your presentation was the illustration of a very difficult yet crucial concept—I refer to the importance of the economic principle of interpretation. I am thinking particularly of your third case, N. When the content of what you said did not fit with the affect nor with what was going on in the transference, you decided to go to where the affect and the transference were. That is a crucial general principle, and you have beautifully illustrated the concept of the eco-nomic principle of interpretation.

I wonder whether you underemphasize the behavioral aspect of projective identification. In other words, the way in which the patient induces the affect in the analyst. It isn't by magic. It is by subtle aspects of the patient's nonverbal behavior, linguistic style, and so forth. That is an interesting issue, I think. I also want to say that I very much agree with your statement about the complexity of defenses, but I wonder, in regard to T, whether what you described as projective identification was perhaps a combination of projective identification and omnipotent control. What is typical, particularly in narcissistic personalities, in terms of omnipotent control, is the effort to control the analyst so that he is neither too good—which would evoke envy—nor too bad—which would evoke deval-uation. Then the patient feels he is losing his money and is dividing himself by being with such a mediocre analyst. So he has to make the analyst as good as the patient, neither better nor worse, and it seems to me that this is more in the nature of omnipotent control. It is a related mechanism but not exactly projective identification.

Finally, I wonder about the idea that a mechanism can be defensive first, and represent a developmental process later. You mentioned that projective identification was first a defense and then could be seen as being the origin of empathy; it is to this that I am referring. Could the sequence not be the other way round, so that normal mechanisms of development and growth eventually become defensive operations? For example, there is the Kleinian notion that splitting is a defensive operation from birth on, but one could think of splitting as first a passive consequence of the separate building up of experiences linked with very positive and very unpleasant affect states. This separate building up can eventually be used for defensive purposes. The relation between defensive processes and developmental ones is very complex, but I do agree with the general concept that these mechanisms can be both defensive mechanisms and mechanisms of growth.

M. *Chayes (The Netherlands).* I want to raise two points, the first clinical and the second more theoretical. The clinical comment is perhaps a bit presumptuous because it concerns an interpretation you gave, Miss Joseph, and you know the patient far better than I do. I had this thought on hearing your interpretation of the last dream of your patient. You spoke of "the feeling in the session," referring to the session before he reported the dream, and I think that your choice of wording is indicative of a shared affective experience, perhaps based upon the idea of a blurring of the distinction between yourself and the patient. It indicates, I think, your willingness and ability to contain affect of a despairing quality which the patient presents in the session. He describes his mother as weak and as someone with whom he could not share such a feeling of despair. Later he reports the dream of the two ships and chooses the ship which is sinking. I wonder if one could not place a more *positive* meaning on his choice of the submerged ship. I mean that perhaps he discovered something new in the previous session, that it was possible to share his affect of despair with someone who did not sink under the burden, who was able to contain this affect. Sharing the experience of drowning—perhaps the tears—and the grief must have great meaning for him, and I wonder whether the symbolism of the sinking ship referred perhaps to a lessening of his anxieties about wishes for fusion. Perhaps he realized that in sexuality it is not necessary that one of the parties be maimed or destroyed by a shared experience. The fact that you did not disappear or were not destroyed, but that he could share the painful affect with you may have been something very positive for him.

My second point is theoretical. I find the concept of the depressive position very valuable, and I think it is linked to something which has not been discussed, namely, the concept of manic defense as it was proposed by Melanie Klein, and also by Winnicott, and seen as reflecting fantasies of omnipotent control over and manipulation of the object, with a concomitant contemptuous devaluation of the object. We must be grateful to the Kleinians for having pointed out, among other things, that triangular object relations begin much earlier than the oedipal phase. Patients who have had fixations due to trauma very early may use primitive defense mechanisms of the sort we see in manic defense. The primitive denial is essential in order to be able to buffer the psychic pain of losing infantile objects. Often one sees in such patients, who at the start show very gross and primitive defenses of this sort, a gradual shift from the use of denial to the use of illusion and fantasy in being able to tolerate the onslaught of grief, jealousy, rage, and so on. If these were not buffered they would be overwhelming.

Jon Sklar (U.K.). I very much enjoyed your clear exposition, Miss Joseph, and want to say something that adds to Dr. Kernberg's last point. In your paper you said very clearly—I quote—"it is frequently difficult to determine whether, at any given moment, projective identification is aimed primarily at communicating a state of mind that cannot be verbalized by the patient or whether it is aimed more at entering and controlling (or attacking) the analyst. Often both aims are present and require consideration." I should like to add something to this. Why are not loving feelings being projected and identified with as well? That is something the patient might also, at a certain stage in his development, want to get rid of. At the end of the paper, when you discussed massive projective identification—I must say I have never understood why it has to be massive, as one never hears about minimal projective identification—you talk about the way, at the beginning of life, the baby has the task of getting into the object in order to get away from pain. But it may also, at the same time, be the task of getting back into the state of love with the object, which has been written about as primary object love.

Ulku Gurisik (U.K.). Having worked with sexual perverts for the last ten years, I want to suggest that in the pervert—I think here of your patient Mr. N—there is also a move against the projective identification. Although such a patient would very much like to be inside the object, there is also an enormous fear of this. I thought that this was possibly expressed in the dream he brought about the finger inside the vagina, when you interpreted the patient's wish to be inside you. Could we not also think, in the light of your emphasis on the point that this patient did not take your interpretation in, that it could also be that the patient is extremely frightened of letting you inside him, afraid that you will engulf him or swallow him completely? It is my impression that in the pervert this fear always goes side by side with the wish to be merged with and to be one with the object.

Betty Joseph. I know that it is impossible and boring if one tries to answer every question. But there are a number of points I want to try to tackle, and I shall start with some comments that Otto Kernberg made. He referred to how often, with very sick patients, one had to work on one's countertransference problems between sessions. He found this a thoroughly healthy thing to do, and I agree with him. But I think it is not only with our very sick patients that we have to do this, but that often those patients who do not appear to be very sick, but are subtly projecting something into us, can make us feel too comfortable or too good or too friendly or too nice. We need to notice these things even more than we notice the more disturbing and disturbed manifestations of some of our patients. If we don't we run the risk of being carried along with an analysis which is a bit "half-cocked," if you know what I mean.

There is also an essential point made by Dr. Kernberg as to the enormous importance, if one is to work with projective identification constructively, of not trying to understand the meaning of everything the patient says. What we have to do—and this is linked with what Joe Sandler says—is to try to get at the feeling, the affect of what is being lived and acted emotionally in the session, rather than getting caught up with the content of what is being said, as if that is the very thing we ought to understand. Sometimes it isn't.

Now I do see with Dr. Chayes that there are other ways of looking at N's dream. I personally do not actually think that when the patient got into the ship that it was due to a shared experience which was being continued in the dream. It is difficult to feel that in the patient's movement toward and away from understanding. The feeling of puzzlement and excitement about getting into the sinking ship did not seem to me to be like a good kind of contact or even fusion, but rather more of a backward movement which could quite quickly be put right, with that patient at that stage of the analysis. The warmth and gratitude he experienced when one could show him this seemed to be the very important thing, because there something good has developed from a relationship with a quite separate me. I think that was where the real progress was needed.

I wasn't quite sure about Dr. Chayes's point about manic defense, but it links with something that Otto Kernberg said. I do think that these highly narcissistic patients, who use projective identification a lot, show an enormous need to remain absolutely, omnipotently in control of the analyst, and this may either be expressed by the projective identification or exist alongside it. This is in a way like a manic defense, but I suspect it is on a more primitive level, that it is more of a schizoid defense. It protects not so much against depression as against all the feelings that would go more with dependence.

Dr. Sklar has made a point about massive projective identification. I meant the term just as I used it. I wasn't referring to anything technical, but was trying to discuss, under the heading of massive projective identification, the kind of projective identification one gets when the patient seems to want to get *totally* inside one. It does not refer simply to a bit of envy or to other more partial aspects, but to the more total phenomenon that we saw in T when he pushed his hand right up the vagina, and nothing could stop him then. That is much more total. I think also of all those children who fall asleep and just cannot be got out of their sleep. These are not *partial* projective identifications but fantasies of being totally inside, and that was what I meant when I was using the word "massive." Of course I agree that loving feelings are also projected and contribute to building a good relationship with the object, but in the example I gave, when I said one has to tease out the different motives for projective identification, I was not at that moment considering teasing out the loving from the more controlling and hostile feelings.

I am sure that Dr. Gurisik is right that T had a great fear of allowing me in because of his tremendously invasive kind of controlling projective identification. I think the fear of letting me in will become clearer and more manageable, more able to be analyzed, when we have got through the current situation in which he absolutely holds me in this kind of balance. Then we will get the fears more clearly.

Joseph Sandler. I want to say just a word about the interesting and controversial question of control. I refer to the degree to which one needs to feel that one is controlling the split-off aspect of oneself or of the internal object when it is located in someone else, as opposed to simply believing it to be there and seeing it there. I am convinced that control is an essential element in projective identification used as a defense, but this point may be worth discussing.

K. König (West Germany). I want to address a problem referred to by Joseph Sandler when he talked about the patient pushing the right buttons in the analyst, and by Otto Kernberg when he referred to the verbal and nonverbal means employed by the patient to make the analyst feel and react in a certain way. I believe that one of the difficulties in accepting the notion of projective identification lies precisely in the fact that we have not explored the interpersonal part of the process of projective identification. It has some mystical quality that makes it difficult for some people to accept the concept. I have been doing research on this for some years, and want to mention two major difficulties I have encountered. One is that for someone trained in psychoanalysis it is very difficult to focus on interpersonal processes, because his main interest has always been intrapsychic. If one wants to observe interpersonal things one has to shift one's focus of attention momentarily from the intrapsychic to the interpersonal. Of course we do that all the time to a certain extent, but it has to be done more if we want to focus on the interpersonal. One of the difficulties we encounter is the problem of differentiating—and such differentiation is important—between the means a patient employs to actualize a particular object relationship, a process which is brought about by verbal or nonverbal action, and his reacting to the transferred object he perceives in the analyst. We have two sets of behavioral phenomena here, and it is sometimes difficult to differentiate them, but I believe that research into this sort of thing may be very rewarding clinically. The reasons for this are twofold. One is that if we understand the processes better we may be able to confront a patient with the way in which he tries to evoke certain feelings in the analyst, thereby aiding the resolution of the transference. Secondly, the differentiation helps us to understand the mechanics of the interaction and thus to contain our countertransference feelings.

M. Shoshani (Israel). I am a little confused about the point raised by Betty Joseph and by Otto Kernberg about projective identification being seen either as a defense or as a developmental process. I should like to have some clarification about this because it seems to me that if we look at it as a developmental process then the analyst would tend to contain it more, to absorb it, and then to process it in such a way that the patient could reintroject it into himself. If the analyst looks at it as a defense, then I think that in the process of analysis it would tend to be interpreted too actively or too intrusively. I noticed this in the first case you presented, that of the four-year-old child. There, though the analyst's interpretation was correct and accurate, it was not quite containing enough. But in your own examples there was much more containment shown. I think it tells us that treating projective identification only as a defense rather than as reflecting developmental processes leads to too quick an interpretation, which is not very "holding" for the patient. I would like to know your reaction to this.

Michael Conran (U.K.).   I am a snapper-up of unconsidered trifles, but as I listen to the questions I begin to wonder whether what I snapped up isn't in some way in tune with other people's feelings. In your paper you say: "if the mother is able to tolerate and contain the child's projections, intuitively to understand and stand its feelings." You meant, I take it, the projections of the child or the infant. But what are these projections? Would you like to put some flesh on those bones? Where do these projections that are intuitively understood by the mother begin, and where do they end? Are they all valued? How do we value them? Are they good things? Are they bad? Is the regurgitation of milk, the smell of which some mothers cannot stand, an instance of projection? Is the caressing of the breast by the child's hand a projection? It seems to me that perhaps the Kleinian position is sometimes in danger of offering itself as a latter-day version of the doctrine of original sin.

Joseph Sandler.   Dr. Sohn, are you going to defend original sin?

Leslie Sohn (U.K.).   I will defend the devil incarnate. Despite the last speaker, I enjoyed the whole paper and the discussion. The paper brought up some points which led to technical considerations about these patients. The patient T epitomizes those patients who are totally dominated by their responses to the pleasure-pain principle, and no interpretation of any of the projective processes is possible until after the preliminary negotiation with the patient about what he feels you are going to do to him. If patients feel they are going to be bitten or scratched they will not listen to the interpretations. Next, what seems to have been forgotten about projective identification is that the sane part of the personality represses the insane part, which operates by splitting and projective identification. So if we look at N's dream after the good sessions and after the good interpretations we have the good ferry boat. Then we have the sinking ship. This seems to me to epitomize both aspects of the patient's personality, in which there is a great enjoyment based on the insane part that operates on the basis of projective identification and prefers to go into the drowning position. It seems to be absolutely clear.

The next point I want to bring up is a question that Otto Kernberg and Betty Joseph have spoken about in terms of timing. If, when dealing with a seriously ill or psychotic patient, one can wait for the understanding to develop, one can make the kind of interpretation that Betty Joseph has made. If you don't get to it immediately with a psychotic patient, but get to it ten minutes later, during the course of the session, then there is no point in using that understanding as an interpretation to your patient. You have to wait until the same situation arises in later sessions, because otherwise the patient will feel you are either mad or omniscient, or the patient will become confused.

I have a question to ask which I cannot answer, and perhaps Betty Joseph can help us with her knowledge of the little girl she spoke about. According to the statement made by the analyst, the child projected everything into the analyst. Why did the child choose that mechanism of projective identification? Why didn't the child become the analyst, completely quiet, cold, and careless, and quite indifferent? Why did it choose that form of putting the experience of cold or whatever it was into the analyst? You said that the child became psychotic; in terms of the diagnostic structure of the child tending toward the psychotic end of the spectrum, would you not expect there to be (and this is in answer to Dr. Sklar) a much more massive form of projection without the ability of the analyst to take over the role?

Roger Dorey (France). I have been very impressed by the presentation we have heard today, and particularly by the clinical aspects presented in Miss Joseph's paper. What was specially interesting is that by giving us such a good insight into the way she works clinically, she also allows us to study carefully the technical and theoretical implications of what she is saying. Joseph Sandler has said that we must be cautious and not simply to take her clinical expertise and swallow it whole, and then become all Kleinian. But the situation is more complicated, and we ought to study very carefully the relationship between the clinical, the theoretical, and the technical. What may be particularly valuable is that Miss Joseph has highlighted the fact that, whatever theoretical beliefs we may have, finally the real value of the theory lies in its relation to practice. Through her linking of theoretical and clinical material we are able to see how she works with all sorts of patients, particularly those with borderline conditions. I would like to suggest that within the field of analysis one can, in a sense, see three kinds of representation: the imaginary, the symbolic, and the realistic. What I mean by the real in this context is that which is not capable of being symbolized, which is at the limit of the analytic field. And what you see in projective identification is really a fantasied object relationship, a living out of a fantasy, a kind of close, mutually returning movement, a mirroring movement. That is not really the same as a relationship based on symbols. It is the living out of a fantasy. If in projective identification we have a living out of an imaginary, fantasy relation, then when an alteration occurs, as it did in patient N, we would have a change from this imaginary relationship to a more symbolic ability to relate. This would use words, for example, and it is another way of perhaps giving a theoretical basis to the clinical work. The last point I will make is that when you spoke about countertransference there is a position in which the analyst is a looker-on, someone outside the whole fantasied relation. Then through the interpretation the analyst can help the patient to get to a more symbolized relationship in which the classical analytic work can proceed.

Betty Joseph.   If I understand Professor Dorey correctly, I would agree that one can look at things from different angles. His last point is an interesting one, in which he draws attention to a movement from a situation in which patient and analyst are apparently caught in a kind of circular situation. However, we would hope that the analyst would be aware of it, and one could say that the movement in analysis would occur when the analyst's interpretations free the patient from being caught in that circular situation, from being caught in a situation of acting out a fantasy in the transference, and moving toward a more symbolic relationship. Then the patient would be aware that words are available to be used to understand things. Would that be one way of seeing it? I mean that what one aims to do is to help one's patient see what is going on in the acting-in which he is unconsciously doing in the transference, and to move toward a state of mind where he can get understanding into that process, and then begin to get an increase in understanding—which should be on a more symbolic level. It is an interesting way of looking at it.

I don't think that I can discuss with any real knowledge the question that Dr. Sohn raises when he asks why the child failed to project herself totally into the analyst. I don't know. I think when she started in treatment we were not sure that she was a fully psychotic case, which in fact she turned out to be. Clearly her defenses, poor as they were, simply did not hold. What interests us at the moment is that in this child there appears to be, in her play, something like a struggle to establish an obsessional neurosis. It will be interesting to see whether such an ill child could establish a neurosis to ward off the underlying psychotic part.

In response to Dr. Shoshani, I do think that as I reported it the work sounds more crude and less subtle than it really is. I think it is not just that the student lacked experience, but rather that the case was so crude to handle. It is extremely difficult to be subtle with a child who is shouting at you, screaming at you, who is throwing things at you or diving under your legs. It becomes very difficult to make subtle interpretations.

I am rather surprised that Dr. Conran feels that I think the only part of a relationship between a mother and a child is projective identification. That isn't how I see the total relationship. I see projective identification as a mechanism. We are left with two issues which are really too big for me to try to handle, but perhaps they will come up again. The first is the issue of how projective identification works. How do our patients get under our skins? How do they find our weak spots? How do they get stuff into us? What are these subtle processes? Maybe one day it would be worth spending more time looking at one small piece of material on one case, and seeing whether some of these things could be teased out, because they really are problems in all our minds. The second big issue, I think, is the question of the relation between defense and developmental processes. To my mind defenses start at the beginning of life. They are defenses which protect the child from feeling overwhelmed with anxiety, whether this comes from the death instinct or from some other source. As the child builds up a warmer and more trusting relationship with his world, these very rigid kinds of defense can lessen and shift away. To my mind one is always getting an interaction between developmental and defensive aspects. I think that Freud was getting at something like this when he discussed the pleasure principle and the reality principle, and suggested that we can begin with how the infant projects into the external world everything that is unpleasant, including parts of himself, and tries to introject into himself the parts that are pleasant. This builds up hallucinatory wish fulfillment. It seems clear that Freud was seeing these primitive defenses, which lessen if the individual develops well. The child or infant will become more able to cope with reality. This is the way that I would see development and defense as going hand in hand.

Chapter 7

Projection and Projective Identification
Developmental and Clinical Aspects

OTTO F. KERNBERG

DEFINITIONS

The term projective identification, introduced by Melanie Klein (1946, 1955) and elaborated by Rosenfeld (1965) and Bion (1967), has suffered the fate of other psychoanalytic concepts in that its meaning has become blurred; it has been used to mean too many different things by too many different people under too many differing circumstances. A recent example is that of Ogden (1979), who, in an attempt to define the mechanism within a strictly clinical context and to dissociate it from any implications of obligatory linkage with Kleinian theory, has stressed its interpersonal in addition to its intrapsychic aspects. I find his contribution helpful, but, unfortunately, in proposing to include under projective identification the therapist's intrapsychic elaboration of what the patient has projected and the therapist's returning to the patient, in the form of an interpretation, a modified or elaborated version of what has been projected, Ogden has broadened the definition of the concept to an extent I think unwarranted. A second disability afflicting the term is its having acquired secondary ideological implications: it has become inextricably linked with the Kleinian theory and is hence viewed with distaste by those who reject that approach.

I have found the phenomenon (as I defined it in 1975) extremely useful clinically, especially when it is considered vis-à-vis the mechanism of

A modified version of this paper has been written for the *Journal of the American Psychoanalytic Association*.

projection. Clinical experience has led me to define projective identification as a primitive defense mechanism consisting of (a) projecting intolerable aspects of intrapsychic experience onto an object, (b) maintaining empathy with what is projected, (c) attempting to control the object as a continuation of the defensive efforts against the intolerable intrapsychic experience, and (d) unconsciously inducing in the object what is projected in the actual interaction with the object.

Projective identification so defined differs from projection, which is a more mature type of defense mechanism. Projection consists of (a) repression of an unacceptable intrapsychic experience, (b) projection of that experience onto an object, (c) lack of empathy with what is projected, and (d) distancing or estrangement from the object as an effective completion of the defensive effort. There is neither empathy with what is projected nor induction in the object of a corresponding intrapsychic experience.

Projection is seen, typically, in the defensive repertoire of patients with neurotic personality organization. In the treatment situation, the hysterical patient who presents fears that her analyst might become sexually interested in her, without any awareness of her own sexual impulses or a parallel communication of such impulses by nonverbal means (so that the "accusation" of the therapist's sexual interest in her occurs within an essentially nonerotic atmosphere) illustrates the same process. Patients with borderline personality organization may use both projection and projective identification, but the latter clearly dominates the patient's defensive repertoire and the transference situation. Patients with psychotic personality organization typically present projective identification as a prevalent defense. Psychotic cases that do show projection—for example, of homosexual impulses that are not consciously experienced in some persecutory delusions, or erotic feelings in patients with no awareness of their own erotic strivings—are much less frequent than the early literature would imply. In short, although projection and projective identification may be present in the same patient, projection is typical of a higher level of functioning, whereas projective identification is typical for borderline and psychotic personality organizations.

I propose that a developmental line leads from projective identification, which is based on an ego structure centered on splitting (primitive dissociation) as its essential defense, to projection, which is based on an ego structure centered on repression as a basic defense. More generally speaking, developmental sequences linking primitive with advanced types of other defensive operations can also be traced. For example, we see a developmental continuum from primitive idealization based on the splitting off of idealized object relations from persecutory object relations, to idealization typical for the narcissistic personality (in which self-idealization, either ego-syntonic or projected, is the counterpart of devaluation), to the idealization typical of neurotic personality organization (which reflects reaction formations against guilt), to, finally, normal idealization as part of the externalization of integrated aspects of the ego ideal. Or else, denial as defined by Jacobson (1957), which is based on dissociation or splitting of contradictory ego states, may be the primitive form of negation, a more advanced mechanism based on repression, a typical neurotic defensive operation. In a still different area, primitive introjection under conditions of lack of differentiation between self- and object representations may be the forerunner of later forms of introjection that are part of the mechanism of selective, partial identifications characteristic of advanced stages of ego and superego development. In short, the prevalence of splitting or repression as a central means of defense would determine whether projective identification or projection predominates.

One important issue that confuses efforts to define projective identification is the question to what extent it is a "psychotic" mechanism. To put the problem another way: to what extent does projective identification imply lack, or blurring, or loss of boundaries between self and object? I believe that projective identification is not necessarily a "psychotic" mechanism, unless the term *psychotic* is used as a synonym for *primitive*, an idea I would reject. When intrapsychic and external object relations occur under conditions of blurring of self- and object representations and lack of differentiation between self and others, such object relations may rightly be called psychotic.

Projective identification may occur with patients having psychotic object relations. When it does, it may represent a last-ditch effort to differentiate self from object, to establish a barrier of a sort between the object and the self by means of omnipotent control. In these circumstances projective identification is the patient's way of trying to avoid a complete loss of self in psychosis. Without recourse to projective identification the patient would lapse into a confusional state in which he or she would no longer be able to know whether aggression, for example, came from the inside or the outside.

In patients with borderline personality organization, whose boundaries between self- and object representations, and between self and external objects, are well differentiated, projective identification has different functions. Here it is the primitive dissociation or splitting of "all good" from "all bad" ego states that the patient attempts to maintain. In patients with borderline personality organization, projective identification tends to weaken the differentiation between self and external objects by producing an "interchange of character" with the object, so that something internally intolerable now appears to be coming from the outside. That exchange between internal and external experience tends to diminish reality testing in the area of the exchange, but the patient maintains a boundary of a sort between the projected aspects and his or her self-experience. In short, projective identification is neither necessarily based on a lack of differentiation between self- and object representations (although it may occur under such conditions), nor does it necessarily cause a loss of differentiation between self- and object representations, although it weakens reality testing.

The clinical observation that interpretation of projective identification in psychotic patients may temporarily increase a patient's confusion and *reduce* his reality testing, whereas interpretation of projective identification in borderline conditions temporarily *increases* reality testing and ego strength are empirical observations that support, in my view, the theoretical conclusions and definitions suggested.

Projective identification, then, is a primitive defensive operation not necessarily linked to psychosis. It predominates in the psychoses, where it is accompanied by loss of reality testing and, from a structural viewpoint, by the loss of boundaries between self- and object representations. In borderline personality organization, projective identification is accompanied by the maintenance of reality testing (structurally underpinned by differentiation of self- from object representations) and permits the use of particular therapeutic techniques to deal with it interpretively, with the result that reality testing and the patient's ego are strengthened. Projective identification plays a relatively unimportant role in the neuroses except when the patient undergoes severe temporary regression; here it is for the most part replaced by projection. In my view, the problems with the definition of projective identification in the literature are related, at least in part, to the different patient populations studied (for example, schizophrenic versus borderline patients), and the failure to differentiate between defensive operations, on the one hand, and the patient's general structural characteristics, on the other.

DEVELOPMENTAL CONSIDERATIONS

If projective identification implies that the subject has the capacity to differentiate between self and nonself, and between an intrapsychic reality and an external one, the subject must have reached a certain level of development before it can be assumed that projective identification is operational. There are currently two very different perspectives from which earliest development has been explored from a psychoanalytic viewpoint. First is the perspective of empirical research on infant development, with its stress on the surprising capacity for very early differentiation between "self" and "object" in the sense of the neonate's clear capacity to place the origin of external stimuli, to carry out cross-modal integration of perceptive qualities of objects, to differentiate the mother's voice and the affective implications of her facial expressions, and so forth (Emde, Kligman, Reich, and Wade, 1978; Stern, 1983). These findings might be used to justify the view that a capacity to differentiate self from objects exists from the earliest weeks of life, and with this, the theoretical possibility that the infant has the capacity to project.

The second perspective for formulating theories of early development is based on the data derived from the transference developments during psychoanalysis and psychoanalytic therapy, particularly the crucial function of manipulation of symbols as the basis for intrapsychic developments.

Granting the possibility that projective identification as a full-fledged defense with all the characteristics mentioned, particularly its interpersonal features, derives from an original stage in which it is only an intrapsychic operation with a predominance of fantasy over actual behavior, the very capacity for fantasy nonetheless requires at least the capacity for symbolization, that is, of some primitive kind of thought processes by which one element stands for another and can be manipulated in the direction of a desired goal.

The differentiation of self from object described by infant researchers may well be "wired in," and reflect constitutionally determined capacities of the central nervous system which do not yet reflect thought processes in the sense of manipulation of symbols, or the subjective awareness of a differentiated self. By the same token, the early activation of complex affective processes, with their neurovegetative, psychomotor, communicative, painful or aversive, and pleasurable or rewarding subjective qualities, may justify a concept of inborn disposition toward and capacity for the experience as well as expression of affects, even if not yet the capacity for symbolic thinking.

I assume that the infant learns when stimulated by extreme pleasure or pain—that is, when he is in a peak affect state. Learning, however, also takes place under different circumstances, with modulated affective conditions, and different consequences. I also assume that very early learning takes place by the infant's associating contiguous stimuli, that one element in a series of stimuli may come to represent the entire series, and that this process is the beginning of the capacity to symbolize. More specifically, when one element of a conditioned series of associations to a peak affect state comes to represent that entire series outside the rigid sequence of associational learning, a basic type of symbolic thinking has been achieved.

In other words, I think that symbolic thinking originates in relation to peak pleasurable and unpleasurable experiences. In this regard, it needs to be stressed that the infant in peak affect states is in a state of particularly motivated attention and thus more susceptible to learning. Empirical research is, however, for methodological reasons, usually carried out only when the infant is in a mild or moderately rewarding as opposed to a negative peak affect state. I assume that learning in these different states does not develop in parallel and that it is the learning that takes place under the impact of both positive and negative peak affects that determines the core nature of the mental representations of self and objects that are established.

Shifting from consideration of the minimal requirements for the assumption of symbolic thinking to that of the development of a subjective sense of self, I have proposed that this development may be conceived as taking place in at least three stages: (a) an earliest state of primary consciousness or subjectivity, first activated during peak affect states and characterized solely by affective experience without any sense of self; (b) a later stage of self-awareness, that is, a reflective awareness of a subjective state that differs from other subjective states; and (c) an integrated sense of self as the basis for a self-reflective awareness of any particular subjective state—the "categorical self" of the philosophers. Self awareness is now not only that of temporarily changing subjective experiences while "a self looks on" but a clear awareness of a continuous entity of a subjective self as something stable against which each subjective state is evaluated.

The earliest stage does not require the capacity for symbolic thinking. The "wired in" capacity for activation of affects and the capacity to associate simultaneous and/or sequential perceptual, psychomotor, neurovegative, and affective experience per se may be all that is present. The second stage is the earliest at which one may assume the process of projective identification to be possible. Only when a particular subjective state is recognized as extremely undesirable in comparison to other subjective states does it make sense to attempt to get rid of it by expelling it onto the periphery of the subjective world.

Projection, by contrast, requires the achievement of a further state of development in which the continuity of self-experience under contradictory emotional circumstances is matched by a clear differentiation between representations of self and of object, and between self and external objects. In fact, strictly speaking, insofar as the organization of the ego typical for borderline personality organization implies differentiated but not yet integrated ego boundaries, and a lack of integration of the self-concept with multiple self-representations alternating in subjective dominance, the conditions for repression as a way of protecting the conscious ego from repressed material are not yet available, and projection per se is not yet operational. Projection, as defined, would require the final integration of the self concept or "categorical self" that is present with neurotic and normal personality organization.

Returning to my formulation of the development of a subjective sense of self, the second stage of development, wherein the infant is capable of comparing different states of self-experience, illuminates the relationships between introjection, projective identification, intersubjectivity (the awareness of the other and of the other's having a subjective experience), and self-experience.

Projective identification may constitute the infant's earliest effort at differentiating self- and object representations under conditions of peak negative affects. Introjection, by contrast, may follow, rather than initiate, the infant's gradual cognitive differentiation of self from object in highly pleasurable states. Such states may gradually blend with the cognitive learning (and differentiation) of non–peak affect experience. The subjective experience of peak pleasurable affect under conditions when memory of different affect states is already available may be accompanied by a self-awareness in its earliest form, without necessarily differentiating self from object in the process. "Intersubjectivity," one might say, is naturally built into the most primitive states of elation activated in infant-mother interactions. Introjection as an active and adaptive process, as well as a defensive one, may therefore originate only later, when "good" self- and object representations have already been differentiated from each other, that is, under structurally quite different circumstances from the original appearance of projective identification. It is possible that projective and introjective mechanisms have a more complex trajectory and less direct relations to each other than has heretofore been assumed. In any case, conditions of extreme pleasure may establish a "good" undifferentiated self-object representation, while absolute unpleasure motivates efforts toward an early escape from and elimination of unpleasure toward the "out there," creating an "all bad" self-object representation in the process.

Projective identification is an attempt, in primitive fantasy, to separate from what is unbearable in order to control it; introjection is an attempt at reunion in fantasy with a loved object. The integration of the self-concept in the context of overcoming splitting processes, and the consolidation of total as opposed to part object relations, may, under normal circumstances, strengthen introjection and diminish projective identification. Under pathological circumstances, however, introjection may become contaminated by projective identification, and vicious circles may ensue that perpetuate predominantly intolerable, aggressively invested unconscious object relations. The vicissitudes of self and object differentiation and the cognitive support to the differentiation of ego boundaries in the course of development may contribute to establishing the structural landmark of reality testing that further influences the destiny of projective identification: its transformation into projection.

Accordingly, projection may be conceived as a "healthier," more adaptive outcome of projective identification, at least at early stages of integration of the self-concept and consolidation of repressive barriers. Eventually, of course, projection has maladaptive consequences because of the distortion of external reality it implies.

Projective identification fosters differentiation under conditions of unpleasurable peak affect states. Insofar as what is attributed to the "out there" is something originally and painfully experienced as subjective awareness, self-reflectively rejected, projective identification also establishes by the same token "intersubjectivity." Projective identification, one might say, assures the capacity of empathy under conditions of hatred, in a parallel way to the development of empathy as a concomitant of the differentiation between self- and object representations under pleasurable peak affect experiences that leads to introjection. In this latter sense, empathy as an early mode of concordant arousal to other people's affective expressions may correspond to an originally "wired-in" disposition and most probably predates the development of self in a "categorical" sense. Empathic arousal is empirically observable at times of mild or moderate positive affective arousal or in states of relative affective quiescence (Hoffman, 1978). It intensifies under conditions of pleasurable peak affective experience and, we may assume, deepens when introjection of the "good" object consolidates a rich intrapsychic representation of the object. This advanced stage of empathic identification corresponds to the unconscious process of introjective identification and is the basis for the positive, libidinal aspects of intersubjectivity.

Projective identification, by contrast, although originating in a primitive empathy with what is projected, attempts to dissociate what is projected from the self-experience and thus operates against the establishment of empathy in the ordinary sense of the word. Eventually, however, the integration of love and hatred, of positive and negative self-representations into an integrated self, and of object representations into integrated conceptions of others facilitates the toning down of projective identification, and determines the capacity for maintenance or reestablishment of empathy under conditions of predominance of aggression. The tolerance of aggression toward the object facilitates the internalization of the object when it is experienced as aggressive, thus reactualizing the empathic origin, we might say, of projective identification.

CLINICAL MANIFESTATIONS AND TECHNICAL APPROACHES

The analyst listening with an analytic attitude to the patient depends on two sources of information: first, the direct communication of subjective experience by the patient talking as freely as he can about what is going on in his mind. Under ordinary transference developments, the analyst may experience transitory concordant and complementary identifications in his emotional reactions to the patient, that is, more or less "realistic" reactions to the transference that blend naturally with the analyst's cognitive understanding. The analyst is thereby able to expand his knowledge of the subjective world communicated by the patient by means of language, to empathize with it, and to transform his own understanding into interpretive formulations with a significant degree of internal freedom.

Second, the patient may communicate by means of his nonverbal behavior or may use words not as communication but as a means of action, a direct expression of unconscious material and the defenses against it. While all patients express significant information by nonverbal means, the more severe the character pathology the more nonverbal behavior predominates. Here projective identification is usually employed in modeling the nonverbal aspects of the patient's communication, diagnosable through the analyst's alertness to the interpersonal implications of the patient's behavior and to the activation in himself of powerful affective dispositions reflecting what the patient is projecting.

When verbal communication of subjective experience predominates, projective identification is less evident, less easily diagnosed by the analyst because of its subtle manifestations, but more easily handled interpretively if the analyst preserves his internal freedom for fantasy about the patient and does not suffer from undue countertransference reactions in a restricted sense (that is, unconscious transferences to the patient or his transference).

By contrast, patients with severe character pathology who unconsciously attempt to escape from an intolerable intrapsychic reality by projective identification onto the analyst make it easier for the analyst to diagnose this phenomenon and yet more difficult to interpret it. For the patient typically resists the analyst's efforts at interpretation because of the dread of what had to be projected in the first place. Under certain extreme conditions, for example, in the case of aggressive infiltration of the pathological grandiose self or "malignant narcissism," the patient's capacity to accept the interpretation of projective identification may be strained to the limit.

The following clinical vignettes illustrate the activation of projection and projective identification and their technical management.

Case One

A woman in her early twenties, who started her psychoanalysis suffering from an hysterical personality, consistent inhibition of orgasm in intercourse with her husband, and romantic attachments in fantasy to unavailable men, expressed the fantasy that I was particularly sensual, in fact, "lecherous," and might be attempting to arouse her sexual feelings toward me so as to obtain sexual gratification from her. She said she had heard I came from a Latin American country, that I had written about erotic love relations. Furthermore she thought I had a particularly seductive attitude toward the women working in the office area where I saw her. All this she viewed as justifying her fears. She expressed the fantasy that I was looking at her in peculiar ways as she came to sessions, and that I probably was trying to guess the shape of her body underneath her clothes as she lay on the couch. Initially she had been reluctant to speak openly about these fears, but my interpreting her fearfulness of my rejecting her if she expressed her fantasies about me openly led to a gradual unfolding of this material. Actually her attitude was not seductive: on the contrary, there was something inhibited, rigid, almost asexual in her behavior and very little eroticism expressed in her nonverbal communications. My emotional reactions and fantasies about her had a subdued quality, contained no erotic element, and I concluded that she was attributing to me her own repressed sexual fantasies and wishes. In other words, this typical example of a neurotic transference illustrates the operation of projection, with little activation of countertransference material either in a broad sense (the sum total of the analyst's realistic reaction to the transference, to issues in the patient's life, and his own), or in the restricted sense (of the analyst's emotional reaction derived from unconscious transferences to the patient to be diagnosed only by the analyst's analytic exploration of himself).

A year later, the patient had changed significantly. Her fear of my sexual interest in her had led to her disgust of the sexual interest that older men have for younger women, the discovery of features of her father in such disgusting, lecherous older men, the discovery that her romantic attachments in fantasy were toward men she perceived as unavailable, and that she was afraid of sexual excitement with such previously unavailable but now potentially available men. Her recognition that sexual excitement was associated with forbidden sexual relations opened up the gradual awareness of her defenses against sexual excitement in the relation with me, and led to a decrease in the repression and projection of sexual feelings in the transference, as well as to the emergence of direct oedipal sexual fantasies about me.

At one point the patient expressed quite openly fantasies of a sexual affair with me, concretely expressed as fantasies of a secret trip to Paris. I found myself responding to these fantasies with an erotic response to the patient, including a fantasy that I, in turn, would enjoy a sexual relation with her marked by my breaking all conventional barriers. I would thus provide her as a gift the fullest acknowledgment of her specialness and attractiveness. In other words, in my transitory emotional response to what were very openly expressed oedipal wishes and correspondingly seductive behavior in the transference, there was activated in me the complementary attitude of a fantasied, seductive oedipal father. However, neither projection nor projective identification were operative here: the patient's sexual impulses were ego-syntonic, there was no effort on her part to control me in order to protect herself against such threatening sexual impulses, and in my response I could maintain empathy with her central subjective experience.

It should come as no surprise that a little later the patient became very angry because of my lack of response to her sexual feelings; by the same token, she felt teased and humiliated by me. This led to our exploration of her anger with a teasingly seductive, and as she experienced it, rejecting father. In this neurotic personality structure, the predominance of communication by verbal means of an intrapsychic experience led to the activation of a complementary identification in a transference relationship relatively free of more primitive defensive operations, particularly of projective identification. Repression and projection were dominant defenses, in addition to other typical neurotic defenses such as intellectualization, reaction formations, and negation.

Case Two

A woman in her late twenties suffered from a narcissistic personality disorder with overt borderline functioning, that is, with general lack of impulse control, of anxiety tolerance, and of the capacity for sublimatory channeling. She also suffered from periodic severe depressive reactions with impulsive and severe suicidal tendencies that had already motivated several hospitalizations. She had recently been discharged from the hospital where I had seen her as an inpatient and was continuing in psychoanalytic psychotherapy with me, three sessions a week. She was a physically attractive woman, although staff thought her cold, haughty, and distant. She alternated between periods when she grandiosely and derogatorily dismissed all who tried to help her, and other times when she experienced feelings of inferiority and deep despair.

She had a long history of chaotic relations with men. She became infatuated with men she admired and thought unavailable, but any man interested in her she treated with contempt. She considered herself a "free spirit," thought that she had no sexual inhibitions but rather was very open in expressing her sexual wishes and demands, and maintained simultaneous relationships with several men when that facilitated her social life and provided her unusual experiences or benefits. Yet she was basically honest in her dealings with all these men, and gave no history of antisocial behavior.

Her mother was a dominating, controlling, intrusive woman who, stemming from a relatively humble background, had used her strikingly attractive daughter from early childhood on as a source of gratification for herself, and who (in the patient's perceptions) had no interest in the patient's internal life other than in what reflected on herself as her mother. The father was a successful businessman whom the patient described as a stunningly attractive, sexually promiscuous man who died suddenly of illness during the patient's adolescence. Because of his intense involvement with his business as well as his many affairs, he was practically unavailable to his daughter.

The patient had originally requested that I see her, motivated by the fact that I was the director of the hospital. But when I became her psychotherapist, she felt initially triumphant only to quickly express doubts about whether she wanted to continue in treatment with me.

During the following episode, several weeks after discharge from the hospital and while she was resuming her graduate studies, she expressed strong doubts whether to continue in psychotherapy with me in the "little town" where I treated her, which, as she put it, would totally destroy her motivation and interests because of its ugliness, provincialism, lack of stimulation, and horrible climate. She described the excitement of life in San Francisco or New York, "the only two livable cities in this country," and raised questions about my professional insecurity, reflected, as she saw it, in my remaining in such a small town.

She came to the session elegantly dressed and told me about a former friend, now a prominent lawyer in San Francisco, who had invited her to live with him, an offer she said she was seriously considering. She went on to describe her current lover, whom she had now decided to drop, as ridiculously unattractive in bed. She commented that he was a nice but average person, without subtlety or refinement, inexperienced in bed, and poorly dressed. She then said that her mother had raised the question, after seeing me for the first time, whether her daughter wouldn't benefit more from a therapist who was younger and more energetic, and who could be firm with her: I had impressed her mother as friendly, but plain and insecure.

I asked her what her thoughts were about her mother's comments, and she said that her mother was a very disturbed person but at the same time very intelligent and perceptive. She then smiled apologetically and said that she did not want to hurt my feelings, but that I really dressed in a provincial way and lacked the quiet yet firm sense of self-assurance that she liked in men. She also said that she thought I was friendly but lacked intellectual depth; she also expressed a sense of concern over the extent to which I would be able to tolerate her being open with me. She sounded friendly enough, and it took me a few minutes to recognize the condescending note infiltrating that friendliness.

The patient then went on to talk about plans for meeting her friend in San Francisco. She considered the possibility that he might fly here to visit her before that, and she had some ideas about how to make his brief stay in town an attractive experience in "cultural anthropology," namely, the study of a small-town culture.

As the patient continued talking, I experienced a sense of futility and dejection. Thoughts crossed my mind about the many therapists this patient had had before coming to our hospital, about the general description of her, conveyed to me by several of these therapists, as incapable of committing herself to a therapeutic relationship. I now thought that she was probably incapable of maintaining a therapeutic relationship with me, and that this was the beginning of the end of her therapy. I felt like giving up, that I really would not be able to go beyond the well-organized surface layer of the patient's comments. I suddenly had the thought that I was having difficulties in thinking precisely and deeply, exactly as the patient had just said. I also felt physically awkward, and experienced empathy with the man with whom the patient had just had an affair, whom she had dismissed with derisory comments about his sexual performance.

It was only in the final part of this session that I became more fully aware that I had become just one more devalued man, and that I stood for all the men who had first been idealized and then rapidly devaluated. I now remembered the patient's expressed anxiety in the past over my not taking her on as my patient, her desperate sense that I was the only therapist who could help her, and the intense suspicion she had expressed in the first few sessions that I was interested merely in learning all about her difficulties only then to dismiss her, as if I were a collector of rare "specimens" of patients and had basically a derogatory attitude toward them. I decided there was an act of revenge in the patient's devaluation of me, the counterpart of her sense in the past that I would assert my superiority and devalue her. And it then came to mind that I was also feeling much the way she had described herself feeling when she felt inferior and in despair, when she felt stupid, uneducated, incapable of living up to the expectations of the brilliant men she had been involved with in the past. And I recognized in her behavior toward me the attitude of quiet superiority and subtly disguised devaluation with which the mother, as the patient had described her, made fun of her because of the inappropriate nature of the men she selected for herself.

The session ended before I could sort out all these thoughts, and I believe I may have conveyed to the patient the impression of being both silent and slightly dejected.

The continuation of the same themes in this patient's communications in the next session included plans for meeting the desirable man from San Francisco, the final stages of the dismissal of her current lover, and further derogatory comments about the "small town." In this connection, I also realized that she had even managed to activate in me, during the last session, whatever ambivalence I myself experienced about the town in which I lived. Only now did I become aware that this town also stood for me in the transference, that the town and I also represented her own devalued self-image projected onto me, while she was identifying with the haughty superiority of her mother. I now thought that it was likely that she was both enacting one aspect of her grandiose self, namely, the identification with her mother, while projecting onto me the devalued aspects of herself and, at a different level, submitting to her mother's efforts to destroy her efforts to get involved with a man who might care for her. Now a memory came back to me, one that had been temporarily obliterated in the previous session, regarding her earlier expressed fears that I would try to prevent her from leaving town because of my own needs to keep an interesting patient, and my earlier interpretation of this fear that it represented her view of my behaving like her mother, an interpretation she had accepted in the past.

I now said that her image of me as intellectually slow, awkward, and unattractive, "stuck" in an ugly town, was the image of herself when she felt criticized and attacked by her mother, particularly when her mother didn't agree with her choice of men, and that her attitude toward me had the quiet superiority, the surface friendliness, and yet subtle devaluation that she experienced so painfully coming from her mother. I also said that in activating the relationship with her mother with an inversion of roles she might also be very frightened that I would become totally destroyed and that she might have to escape from the town to avoid the painful disappointment and sense of loneliness that would come with this destruction of me as a valued therapist. The patient replied that she could recognize herself as she would feel in other times in what I was describing, and that she had felt dejected after our last session. She said she felt better now, and could I help her make the visit of the man from San Francisco a success, so that he would not depreciate her because she was now in such an unattractive place? She now reverted to a dependent relationship with me, practically without transition, while projecting the haughty, derogatory aspects of herself as identified with her mother onto the man from San Francisco.

This case illustrates a typical activation of projective identification, including the projection of an intolerable aspect of herself, the behavioral induction of the corresponding internal attitude in me, the subtle control exerted over me by her derogatory dismissal and self-assertion that kept me temporarily imprisoned in this projected aspect of herself, and her potential capacity for empathizing with what had been projected onto me because, at other points, it so clearly corresponded to her self-representation. This example also shows that what was projected was a self-representation, although, at a different level, it may also correspond to other objects onto whom such a self-representation had been projected in the past, while the patient activated a specific object representation that, in this case, had become a constituent of a pathological grandiose self-structure. My countertransference reaction illustrates a complementary identification and, beyond that, my temporarily getting "stuck" in it, what Grinberg (1979) has designated as "projective counteridentification."

Case Three

This patient, a business manager in his early forties, presented a paranoid personality with borderline personality organization, a history of brief psychotic episodes under the effects of alcohol, brief hospitalizations for such psychotic episodes, and dissociated homosexual longings that became ego-syntonic only when he was intoxicated. He suffered from severe social and work inhibitions, and impulsive rage attacks had on various occasions threatened his work situation and social life. He also presented severe sexual inhibitions in heterosexual encounters, frequent episodes of impotence, and a chronically suspicious, distrustful attitude that interfered both with opportunities for sexual intimacy and with his interpersonal relations in general.

He was the oldest of several brothers born to a pharmacist who had become prominent in the social life of the small town where they lived, a powerful, irate, extremely demanding and sadistic man who punished his children severely for minor misbehaviors. The patient's mother was completely submissive to his father, and although she professed to love her children, she never went out of her way to protect them from the father's rages. She was shy and socially withdrawn, and left the care of her children to several of her older unmarried sisters who lived in the household and acted as maids and "surveillance agents" for the father, and who treated his children with particular strictness. The patient vividly recalled puritanical attitudes about sex. The patient felt that his younger siblings were able to escape from what he considered the dreadful atmosphere of his home, while he, as the eldest son, could not escape the constant control of his father. Against his father's wishes he went into a large farming equipment business, and because of his severe personality difficulties never managed to advance beyond middle level managerial positions, in spite of an excellent academic background, unusually high capacities in the field of marketing analysis, and a better education than several colleagues who had been promoted above him.

In the transference the patient oscillated between periods of intense fears and suspicions about me perceived as a sadistic father and other times of intense idealization of me linked to homosexual impulses, thus illustrating typical splitting mechanisms. In the course of the first two years of treatment I had interpreted to him his activation of these emotionally opposite relations to me as the alternative enactment of two aspects of the relation to his father, namely, an unconscious identification with his mother in submitting sexually to an idealized father who would provide love and protection and rage against his sadistic father. He had gradually began to tolerate his intense ambivalence toward his father and had begun to talk quite openly about his murderous wishes toward him. The following episode took place in the third year of his treatment.

The patient had made the acquaintance of a lady working in the large complex of psychiatric institutions with which I was associated. For the first time he had dared to become active in pursuing a relationship with a woman whom he found physically attractive and who was socially and intellectually at his level. In the past he had felt safe only in relations with prostitutes or in distant, asexual relations with a few female friends. At any sign of involvement with a woman he valued he would quickly break away, intensely suspicious of the woman's intentions toward him and afraid that he might be impotent. On several occasions he had expressed the fantasy that I would feel unhappy over his getting involved with anyone who worked in an institution related to the one I worked in, and expressed the suspicion that I would approach her to warn her against him and interfere with the developing relationship. I had begun to interpret this as an expression of oedipal fantasies, commenting to him that, in his mind, I was the owner of all the women in that extended psychiatric "society," that his sexual approach to them was forbidden by me as the father, and that, in his fantasy, he might be severely punished. I also linked this fantasy to his fears of impotence with a woman who would seem fully satisfactory to him. A few days after this interpretation the patient came in, livid with rage.

He started by saying that he felt like punching me in the face. He sat down in a chair at the greatest distance from me and asked me for a full explanation. When I asked him, an explanation about what, he became even further enraged at my "playing innocent." After several moments of mounting tension, during which I became genuinely afraid that he might hit me, he finally explained that he had spent an evening with this lady, that he had asked her whether she knew me and had learned that, indeed, she did. When he then pressed her for information about me, she became very reticent and asked him "ironically," as he saw it, whether he was a patient of mine. He then confronted her with what he considered a fact, namely, that she had known all along that he was a patient of mine. Then she became even more distant and finally ended the evening by suggesting that they had better "cool" their relationship.

The patient now accused me of having called her, of telling her all about his problems, of warning her against him, and of causing the end of the relationship. My effort to connect this with my past interpretations of his experience of me as owner of all the women of the institutional complex and jealous guardian of my exclusive rights over them further heightened the patient's rage. He accused me of dishonestly misusing my interpretations to deny the facts and to put the blame on him for the breakdown of the relationship. He now focused on my dishonesty—he could tolerate my prohibitions but not my dishonesty. He demanded that I confess that I had forbidden her to enter into a relationship with him.

The patient's rage was so great that I was not at all sure he would not physically attack me. I was really in a dilemma: either I acknowledged as true the patient's mad construction or insisted that what he was saying was false, thereby risking being physically assaulted. Earlier doubts about whether the patient's paranoid traits really permitted an analytic process added to my uneasiness.

Taking a deep breath, I told the patient that I did not feel free to talk as openly as I would want to, because I was not sure whether he could control his feelings and not act on them. Could he assure me that, however intense his rage, he would refrain from any action that might threaten me or my belongings? The patient seemed taken aback by this question and asked me whether I was afraid of him. I said that I did fear a physical attack by him and told him that I felt I could not work under these conditions. He would therefore have to assure me that our work would continue within the context of verbal discourse rather than physical action or I would not be able to continue working with him in this session.

The patient then smiled and said I did not need to be afraid, he just wanted me to be honest. I said that if I answered him honestly he might get very angry at me, and could he assure me that he would be able to control his rage? He said he could. I then said that while I knew the lady, I had not talked with her during the entire duration of his treatment, and that his assertions were a fantasy that needed to be examined analytically. The patient promptly became enraged with me again, but now I no longer felt afraid of him.

After listening to his detailed and angry presentation of all the reasons that had convinced him that I was involved in her rejection of him, I interrupted him to say that I believed he was absolutely convinced that I had stopped her relationship with him. I then added that he was now in the painful position of having to decide whether I was lying to him, or whether I was equally convinced that he was wrong and that we were therefore involved in a mad situation in which one of us was aware of reality and the other not, and it could not be decided which of us was where. The patient grew visibly more relaxed, and said he believed my saying I was not lying. He then added that, for some strange reason, all of a sudden the whole issue seemed less important to him. He said he felt good that I had been afraid and had confessed as much to him.

A rather long silence ensued, in the course of which I sorted out my own reactions. I experienced a sense of relief because the patient was no longer attacking me, a feeling of shame because I had shown him my fears of being physically assaulted, feelings of anger because of what I perceived as his sadistic enjoyment of my fear without any compunction over that enjoyment, and an intolerance of his enjoyment of that sadistic acting out. I also felt that the whole relationship with the woman seemed, all of a sudden, less important, which I found puzzling but could not explain to myself further.

I then said that a fundamental aspect of the relationship with his father had just taken place, namely, the enactment of the relationship between his sadistic father and himself as a frightened, paralyzed child, in which I had taken the role of the child and he the role of his rageful father secretly enjoying his intimidation of his son. I added that my acknowledgment of my fear had diminished his own sense of humiliation and shame at being terrorized by his father, and the fact that it was safe to express rage at me without destroying me made it possible for him to tolerate his own identification with his enraged and cruel father. The patient then said that perhaps he had frightened the woman because of his inquisitorial style in asking about me, and that his own suspiciousness about her attitude toward him while she acknowledged that she knew me might have contributed to driving her away.

This case illustrates projective identification being employed at an almost psychotic level. It is of interest to point out that initially the patient used projection in attributing to me a behavior that did not resonate at all with my internal experience. Then, in attempting to force me into a false confession, he regressed from projection into projective identification, activating the relationship with his father with reversed roles. In this case, in contrast to the previous one, the violent nature of the projective identification appeared to significantly affect the patient's reality testing, and my efforts to directly interpret projective identification were futile. My acceptance of the complementary identification in my countertransference as a realistic reaction to the transference was, I believe, a less regressive phenomenon in me than the more unrealistic counteridentification mentioned in the previous case. At the same time, I had to initiate my efforts at interpretation by temporarily moving away from a position of technical neutrality, establishing a condition for continuing the session that implied a restriction of the patient's behavior. Only then could I deal with the projective identification itself by establishing first a clear boundary of reality or, more specifically, by spelling out the nature of the "incompatible realities" that now characterized the analytic situation. I think the clarification of incompatible realities as a first step to facilitate the patient's tolerance of a "psychotic nucleus" in his intrapsychic experience is an extremely helpful way of dealing with such severe regressions in the transference. By the same token, establishing the boundaries of reality also reestablishes the analyst's internal freedom to deal with his countertransference reactions. This technique must be differentiated from countertransference acting out, a difference that at times is rather hard to detect.

FURTHER CONSIDERATIONS ON TECHNIQUE

I have tried to present illustrations of my approach to the interpretation of projection and projective identification. As part of this technique, the analyst must diagnose in himself the characteristics of the self- or object representation projected onto him, so that he can interpret to the patient (a) the nature of this projected representation, (b) the motives for the patient's intolerance of that internal experience, and (c) the nature of the relationship between that projected representation and the one enacted by the patient in the transference at that point. The persecutory nature of what is projected in projective identification typically induces fears in the patient of being criticized, attacked, blamed, or omnipotently controlled by the analyst. Systematic interpretation of this secondary consequence of the interpretation of projective identification may facilitate working through over a period of time.

The analyst's intrapsychic experience when severe forms of projective identification are activated may disturb or help the analytic process. The analyst's firm maintenance of technical neutrality, his lack of communication of the countertransference to the patient, and his refraining from setting up parameters of technique not originally planned for this particular treatment may all facilitate the analyst's internal freedom for fantasying during the sessions with the patient as well as outside the sessions, gradually clarifying and working through his countertransference reactions and developing alternative hypotheses and strategies to interpret the transference under such trying conditions. For the analyst to be excessively preoccupied with severely regressed patients outside the treatment hours may be healthy, not necessarily neurotic. In fact I believe that, under conditions of severe regression in the transference and a strong predominance of activation of projective mechanisms, a significant part of the analyst's working through of his own countertransference reactions may have to occur in work outside the hours.

When, as can happen, borderline personalities with dominantly narcissistic and paranoid features undergo a temporary psychotic regression in the transference, it may be necessary for the analyst to stop interpreting and to clarify in great detail the immediate reality of the treatment situation, including asking the patient to sit up and to discuss with him in great detail everything that has led to his present paranoid stance, a course suggested by Rosenfeld (1978). The analyst should absorb the patient's projective identification without interpreting it for the time being, acknowledging empathy with the patient's experience without accepting responsibility for it, thus demonstrating the analyst's capacity to tolerate the patient's aggression without counteraggression or crumbling under it, an application of Winnicott's "holding" function. The analyst should consistently interpret projective identification in an atmosphere of objectivity that provides a cognitive "containing" function—Bion's approach. Finally, the analyst should set limits to acting out that may threaten the patient or the analyst's physical integrity (if such limits are objectively required), test the extent to which reality testing is still maintained in the interaction (with the assumption that interpretation cannot proceed before a common boundary with reality has been reestablished), and analyze "mutually incompatible realities."

This last method includes a full acknowledgment and spelling out of the patient's current experience, of the analyst's experience of the situation (which may be totally incompatible with the patient's), and the proposal that these mutually incompatible experiences constitute a valuable frame of reference for the analysis of affective experience under the condition of the potential "madness" of one of the participants without prejudice as to where to locate this madness. This method, of value under some rather extreme circumstances, facilitates, in my experience, the maintenance of an interpretive approach based on consistent technical neutrality, a demystification of the patient's regressive transference experience, and, eventually, a potential tolerance on the part of the patient of the "mad" part of his mind.

At times the analyst's emotional dissociation from the situation, his temporary "giving up" on the analytic experience, may provide a distancing device that may detoxify the therapeutic relationship, but at the cost of potential disruption of the treatment, or a temporary or permanent going "underground" of primitive transferences, a safety valve, therefore, that has its risks and dangers as well as its advantages.

These various techniques are largely compatible with each other, but there are differences in emphasis. My own approach utilizes the application of Bion's "containing" function (1967), Winnicott's "holding" function (1958), Rosenfeld's understanding of the nature of severely regressive transferences in the case of narcissistic character pathology (1971, 1975, 1978), and the technique I described to clarify the reality situation before further attempts at interpretation of projective identification under certain regressive conditions.

I believe, however, that Bion's avoidance of the analysis of countertransference issues with severely regressed patients, his assumption that the concept of countertransference should be maintained in its restricted definition, and therefore as an indication of pathology in the therapist, impoverishes the analyst's openness toward the total field of countertransference reactions. Bion (1974, 1975), particularly in the Brazilian lectures, conveys both an exquisite sensitivity to severely regressive transferences and a puzzling lack of concern for the patient's reality situation, which may be the counterpart of his deemphasis of countertransference. I believe that concern for the patient implies commitment to him, and commitment makes the analyst vulnerable to countertransference in a broad sense.

My approach to the confrontation of the patient with incompatible views of reality may be in contrast to Rosenfeld's recommendation (1978) for a temporary abandonment of a confronting and interpretive stance with severely paranoid regressions. My paper illustrates how useful I have found Racker's contributions (1968) to the analysis of countertransference and Grinberg's elaboration and expansion of these views (1979).

To conclude, projective identification is a dominant but not exclusive mechanism involved in the activation of primitive object relations and defenses against them in the regressive transferences of patients with borderline personality organization, and of relatively less importance in patients with neurotic personality organization. Projective identification is a fundamental source of information about the patient and requires an active utilization of the analyst's countertransference responses in order to elaborate the interpretation of this mechanism in the transference.

Chapter 8

Discussion of Otto F. Kernberg's Paper

Joseph Sandler. We have been treated to an extremely clear presentation by Dr. Kernberg, one which links theory to the clinical situation in a remarkable way. The paper raises a number of questions, some of which have been touched on in the previous discussions. One of these relates to the problem of whether we should conceive of only bad or unwanted aspects of the self being projected in projective identification. But what I am thinking of in particular are the idealized qualities that one normally strives for. One could hardly call these "unwanted" aspects of the self, yet it is very common indeed that one lives through another person the self as one would like it to be. This is what Anna Freud referred to when she discussed altruistic surrender in *The Ego and the Mechanisms of Defense* in 1936, and I think it is a very important aspect of our relationships in general. It certainly comes into the analytic situation when the "ideal" wished-for aspects of oneself are not only projected onto the analyst, but the analyst is in fact nudged into fulfilling that role—of course some analysts are more ready to do this than others.

The question also arises of the very interesting distinction made by Dr. Kernberg between projective identification as a primitive mechanism and projection as a more mature one. If I understand him correctly, in projection the boundaries between self and object are maintained, while projective identification, as he describes it, involves very fluid boundaries. Dr. Kernberg has had to deal with the very tricky problem of answering the question of how one puts something outside oneself even before the boundary between self and other, between self and object has been created. I think that he does show how the primitive projective identification represents the infant's attempt to adapt in order to get a better feeling in himself, and how in doing this boundaries get created. It is very plausible to think of a to-and-fro process of "putting out." The boundaries are not yet solidly established but the infant is attempting their establishment. And obviously when experiences return into one's own rudimentary self-representation they get pushed out again, and clearly this must help in the establishment of boundaries. Betty Joseph has made much the same point.

We then come to the question of whether the projective identification that we see in our clinical work and have heard about in the cases described so far is the same as the very primitive projective identification Otto Kernberg has described. I think there must be a case for distinguishing between the two. There may be a danger that one might fall into what I would call the precursor fallacy, the fallacy of considering the precursor to a phenomenon as being essentially the same as the phenomenon itself. I think that the precursor projective and introjective processes that have been described might not really deserve to be put under the same heading as the mechanism of projective identification, in which there is a very clear knowledge of boundaries. This of course raises the problem of explaining where the feeling of identification with what is projected is located. How does that feeling of identification with what has been got rid of come about? And here we have a very tricky situation because at one level we are identified with what we have disposed of into another person, while at another level we have disidentified ourselves from it. We control it in the person we put it into, and we feel we have got it out of ourselves and it doesn't belong to us, but at the same time we need to know that it is a part of ourselves that we have got rid of. This needs some clarification.

Otto Kernberg has given special emphasis to projective identification as a psychotic mechanism, and of course we do at times see the regressive breakdown of boundaries in psychotics. We may then see something which is very similar to early projective identification of the sort that has been described. But I do think that projective identification as a mechanism is a very normal phenomenon indeed. We see it in all relationships which are held together by the cement of idealization—as for example in living through the other person.

My final comments relate to the question of transference, and they have been stimulated by all the papers we have heard so far. We have all been taught (and we teach) that transference is in one form or another a repetition of the past which is inappropriate to the present. At the same time we also tend to consider as transference all the displacements between self and object which occur in the here-and-now of the analytic situation which are not necessarily repetitions of the past. Of course it is much easier for the Kleinians to deal with this problem because they bring the past so much closer to the present, but there are some of us—and I think Otto Kernberg and I are probably at one in this—who see a long developmental process occurring through childhood in which there are great changes in the internal world, with tremendous shifts in the representations of self and object during development, although there are many things that are constant as well. So we may see our patient, in what we would call transference, defensively putting something into the analyst, defensively reversing things in a way we might call projective identification. This mechanism, together with others, including all the different varieties of projection or identification, seems to some extent to be autonomous. Many functions become autonomous during development, and I think that the capacity to projectively identify certainly does become an autonomous function, and is used as such in the present. It is not simply a repetition of the past, although of course it has a history. Otto Kernberg has taken the relatively recent emphasis on the object relationship aspect of motivation and has applied this to his clinical material through the further step of interpreting transference in terms of shifts between self- and object representations. In the transference interpretations which reflect this there is little or no reconstruction of the past. And this leads us to the very interesting problem, which has preoccupied many of us, of the role of reconstruction in our interpretations. I think that the emphasis on reconstruction has lessened. We are perhaps more interested in what is happening between us and the patient in the present, and this is correlated with a shift in the meaning of transference.

W. W. Meissner. I was very stimulated by Dr. Kernberg's talk and am impressed by the very significant degree of congruence of our thinking. I was amazed at the degree to which Betty Joseph's presentation, except perhaps for some of her technical formulations, resonated in my mind. Similarly, Dr. Kernberg's paper is very close to my own thinking. Dr. Sandler too has the very bad habit of thinking the same thoughts that I think.

Joseph Sandler. It must be because of projective identification.

W. W. Meissner. It's certainly something. However, I want to comment on two points in Dr. Kernberg's presentation. The first is a distinction that has been somewhat elided in our discussion. It was perhaps a bit too implicit in my own opening comments, and I think that it needs to be refocused. I refer to the distinction between a one-person system and a two-person system. If one looks at the notion of projective identification within a one-person context, what is being implied is a projection from a self-representation to an object representation within the intrapsychic realm of the individual. It has no reference to anything beyond the object representation itself. We can recognize the projection there, but what does it mean to speak of an identification in that context? It seems to me that what we are getting involved in is an attribution, within the object relationship with which the individual identifies, of an aspect of the self recognized within the object. It *becomes* part of the object, so that the self component either totally—Miss Joseph used the word "massive" here—or partially becomes absorbed into the object representation. It is that, I think, which Dr. Kernberg backs away from a little, and the implications can be spelled out fairly specifically. There has to be a loss of ego boundary. There has to be a de-differentiation of representational components, and to my way of thinking this speaks to a quite primitive mechanism. If we shift that over to a two-person context, what on earth are we talking about when we speak of projective identification? The projection is from the subject—we can say into or onto—an object. But now the internalization is not in the same person; it is in the other. We have a completely different kind of situation. I would be very sympathetic to the use of the term projective identification within a one-person system as described. I would not be sympathetic to it in the two-person system, where it comes about that anything that has the character of this interactive exchange, of externalization and internalization, takes place. This is very common in all kinds of interpersonal situations, not only in transference within the analytic situation but in other kinds of human relationships as well. Need we necessarily—can we really—make sense out of a term like projective identification in that context? It becomes a very muddy issue.

There is a related issue Dr. Sandler touched on which I would like to expand. When we think of transference we have to say that it is not always projective. The mechanism of the transference does not always reflect a projection from the inner world of the patient to, let us say, the representation of the analyst. The classic transference in fact was not that. It was based on displacement. One could conceptualize this in representational terms, although theoretically I do not think it is adequately described in only those terms. Then the projective transference would be the weeding out of some content from a self-representation, with that content then being transferred to an object representation. The displacement transference would be transferring material from an object representation to another object representation. A classic paradigm would be the transference of material contained in the object relationship to, let us say, a primary object in the developmental history of the patient, to the representation of the analyst as the new object–transference figure. In either case, patterns of reaction can be generated within the analytic relationship. Dr. Kernberg has discussed at great length ways in which the projective components in the transference can operate without being magical but rather through a set of identifiable processes that have to do with subtle cues, affective communications, behavioral components, and a whole realm of other things that Dr. Kernberg has touched upon. These shape, elicit, induce a reaction in the other person which we can, let us say, describe as an introjection. In the context of a displacement transference similar kinds of processes can take place, so that we cannot argue that whenever such an interactional situation arises we are necessarily dealing with projection. It may not be projection. One cannot justify calling the mechanism projective until we can identify the content of the presumably projected material transferred onto the analyst as a part of the self-representation of the patient. Only when those links have been established can one say that this particular content is projective. The same is true with displacement. When we can identify, for instance, some attribution to the analyst as reflecting a similar experience or attribute derived perhaps from a father figure in the patient's early life, then we can talk about a displacement transference. So when you see a pattern of interaction and the elicitation of a response, countertransference or otherwise, from the analyst, you cannot necessarily say that it is projective without having the evidence that links it to the self-representation. It is even more difficult to attribute this kind of interactive pattern to something like projective identification. If you hold, as I do, that projective identification has its most authentic and validatable meaning within the one-person system you can see how considerable difficulty arises in trying to extend the concept in an excessively flexible fashion.

Otto Kernberg. I will comment on a few points, not so much in order to bring about closure, but rather to illustrate or illuminate differences. I should like to comment first on Dr. Meissner's questions, and then go back to Dr. Sandler's.

Let me say first of all that to think in terms of a one-person system and a two-person system makes me uneasy. This is because, from a modern psychoanalytic perspective, the origin of intrapsychic functioning is to be seen as a diadic situation. This is seen in the child's bliss in the relationship with the mother, even before it is acknowledged or child and mother are differentiated. It makes no difference whether we go with Melanie Klein and Fairbairn or with Winnicott and Mahler. Intrapsychically and in external reality there is an essentially dyadic situation. It is "interpersonal" in that there is no drive without object relationships, nor object relations without drive. All of these separations are artificial, and the defensive operations we are discussing are at first essentially interpersonal. The purely intrapsychic defenses are *advanced* defenses. Omnipotent control, idealization, devaluation, projective identification, splitting, denial (in Edith Jacobson's sense) all have implied interpersonal functions. From a clinical viewpoint, in the very first session with a borderline patient one can see a severe disturbance in the interpersonal situation because of the activation of primitive defenses. With the neurotic patient everything is usually relatively smooth and relaxed at the start, because the defenses are mostly intrapsychic; the interpersonal aspects are minimal. So what looks like a "one-person system" is actually a highly sophisticated, advanced situation. The assumption that psychoanalysis is going "interpersonal" may reflect a confusion between the historical development of our notion of what interpersonality means from the beginning of life, on the one hand, and the fact that, from a developmental viewpoint, the one-person system is a late achievement, on the other. I think that possibly Dr. Meissner is sticking with the one aspect of Jacobson's thinking which I find the least helpful part of her work, namely the definition of introjection and projection. She sees introjection as the change of a self-representation after an object representation, and projection as a change in an object representation after a self-representation. I think these definitions by Jacobson are the only aspect of her work that has little practical relevance, and I say this with full acknowledgment of how directly my own work stems from that of Edith Jacobson.

Moving now to a broader level of psychoanalytic theory, I want to comment on the problem of different motivational systems. It seems to me that nowadays there are, roughly speaking, three psychoanalytic viewpoints in this respect. One is the Sullivanian-interpersonal-Kohutian view. The second is that of classical ego psychology à la New York Psychoanalytic Society, and the third, the object relations approach, which I associate here with Jacobson, Mahler, Klein, Fairbairn, and even Sullivan to some extent. The proponents of the three views differ in terms of their motivational theory, their concept of psychic structure, and their technique. For the culturalists, for Kohut and for Sullivan, what really motivates people are their relations with others, regardless of drives. It is object relations that count, and this leads in practice to the conclusion that aggression is secondary. The result is, I believe, a significant impoverishment of our theoretical view. I am expressing my own bias here, of course. For the traditional ego psychologists, drives—aggression and libido—are there first, and they are only secondarily invested in object relations. That theory of motivation is reflected in a theory of psychic structure, represented by the differentiation of the structure's ego, super-ego, and id. The struggle between aggression and libido is expressed in the interagency conflicts between ego, superego, and id. I see in Dr. Meissner's approach some of that viewpoint. For the object relations theorists the drives differentiate from the very beginning in the context of object relations, and drives and object relations cannot be teased apart. I have a radical viewpoint on this: I think that drives derive from affect states and that originally it is the internalized object relations, under the impact of certain affects, that are organized into both drives and psychic structure. The affects are organized into libido and aggression, and the object relations derived from primitive units of self- and object representations are eventually consolidated into ego, superego, and id. So, for the cultural-ists and Kohut it is actual past relations with objects which get "stuck" in the psychic apparatus, and it is the replaying of these past actual object relations that determines the nature of the transference. Psychic struc-ture is really seen as fixation of past self-objects or of past interpersonal relations, depending on whether you use Kohut or Sullivan.[1]

I come now to one of Dr. Sandler's comments. What do we think transference is? One contemporary conception that is common to all the object relations theories is that—as Melanie Klein has put it—the trans-ference is a repetition of actual relations from the past, of fantasied relations from the past, and of defenses against both. I think that this is also the point that Dr. Sandler stressed—how much is there in the transference that is a defense against the past in contrast to the simplistic view of transference as actual repetition reflected by the Sullivanian or Kohutian approach, and in contrast also to the tendency to tease out "pure" drives and defenses from the internalized object relationships made by traditional ego psychology? I think that the sicker the patient, the more he presents a complex intrapsychic elaboration of past experience. In other words, object relations which developed in the past and, in the course of development, are intrapsychically "scrambled," are eventually activated as present structure. What we have to do in analyzing is to transform present structure through "unscrambling" of intrapsychic genetics before we can get to the real past. The healthier the patient, the more the transference is like the past. The sicker the patient, the more indirect the road, and I think Dr. Sandler was stressing the indirect road,

---

[1] In my view, by contrast, complex intrapsychic transformations distort, reorganize, and consoli-date both structures into the tripartite structure, and affects into the superordinate motivational system of aggression and libido.

the analysis of intrapsychic developments that cannot directly lead to reconstruction. For me reconstruction with severely ill patients comes late in the game, only after a certain degree of integration has taken place.

This leads me to the issue of displacement raised by Dr. Meissner. I must confess that I am not very favorably inclined to the term displacement, because it seems such a general, nonspecific reference to primary process functioning, and I prefer to think of the transference as the unconscious repetition in the here-and-now of relations that were pathogenically fixated in the past. Let me give a very simple example. Let's assume that I have a hole in my sock, and my patient becomes enraged. Why? He doesn't know. He is just enraged that I should have a hole in my sock. I ask him: "What are you so angry about?" The patient has to think, starts rationalizing, and after we analyze his effort to find some rational explanation for something essentially irrational, it turns out that it reminds him of his mother with holes in her stockings, of her neglectful attitude, of the sloppy attitude of his mother. Now this is for me a transference reaction, but it is not projection in a strict sense. It is, first of all, an inappropriate affect and, by the same token, the enactment of an object relation. The fact that he is enacting the relationship with his mother from the past is, as I see it, not simply a displacement, an unconscious repetition. Let us assume that the patient sees a hole in my sock and then thinks that it is not really a sock but that it is a stocking, and has the fantasy that I am wearing a stocking. Let us assume further that below the surface he thinks there is an effeminate attitude in me, and behind that there is a full-fledged fantasy that I have feminine qualities that I am hiding, that I am a closet homosexual. Now this is a projection, because he is attributing to me qualities that I do not have and that he is unconsciously fighting off. That is different from the first case, which is not a projection in any strict sense. But the first case is not a displacement either: it is a complex transference manifestation. The second case is a projection. If, after that, the patient carries out a full projective identification, then we have projective identification in the transference. If you call all transference a projection, so that projection and transference become the same, the subject matter becomes nebulous. I think there are transferences that do not include projection in a strict sense, and that certain transferences don't include projective identification at all. That would be my way of looking at the topic.

Now, what does identification mean in projective identification? It means that one is attributing something to somebody else, then identifying with that person at the same time. This is one use of the term identification, in the sense of knowing how the other person feels. The identification is an expression of "empathy with." The problem we have, of course, is that when we say "identification" we use it to mean many things at the same time. One is "empathy with," and I think that is included in the term projective identification. By the way, let me say that empathy is for me a developmental series. There is a primitive type of empathy based on introjection, there is an empathy based on projective identification, and there is a higher level empathy based upon the tolerance of ambivalence in object relations, a capacity for tolerating love and aggression in oneself, for integrating one's concept of self and integrating one's concept of object, which permits one to develop empathy in depth with others. So we have different developmental levels of empathy, and all of these could be called identification. One could give them different names. Identification is also used in referring to the modification of the self-representation following the internalization of an object representation. It is used to signify a modification of the self at a stage of development in which self and object are well differentiated, in which the identification is only with partial aspects of the object, in contrast to introjection which has been used for the more global internalization of dyadic relations. The point I want to make here is that in my view it would be impossible for me to give you a full and integrated system of definitions of these various terms with which all of us would be happy, because only a common theory can provide such a system. We are not all functioning on the basis of common theories, and therefore we cannot reach that point as yet. As of now, we may have to limit ourselves to defining the more obvious concepts that are clinically relevant, and leave the general system for later.

I want to make one more point regarding the question Dr. Sandler raised about idealization. His first question related to the projection not only of unwanted parts of the self but of idealized wished-for parts. It seems to me that it is preferable to call that mechanism idealization, and again I would think that there is a series of idealization processes ranging from primitive to advanced. The most primitive idealization is that which is the counterpart of persecution, a consequence of the splitting of good and bad. It is the idealization, the Kleinians would say, of the paranoid-schizoid position. In my terminology it would be primitive idealization. Second, there is the idealization in the narcissistic personality, the projection of pathological grandiose aspects of the self, in which there is a destruction of diadic relations leading to a type of idealization which has completely different characteristics. Third, there is the idealization that is a reaction formation because of unconscious guilt; and fourth, there is the idealization described by Chasseguet-Smirgel, the externalization of one's ego ideal onto another person, creating a joint structure, a "bridge" of identification in terms of the common ideal. For me these are developmental sequences of idealization processes and there is an advantage in separating them from the projective series. So we have a series of projective mechanisms and a series of idealization mechanisms, and I think that denial and negation constitute another such series. We have to think of developmental series of defensive operations, which in turn are related to one another in certain frequent constellations.

Joseph Sandler.   I want to make a very brief comment. As far as the interpersonal is concerned, I think that Sullivan and his immediate followers did not put any stress on the internal world of the individual, on the object relationship to the introject. One can be motivated, I believe, by interpersonal dialogues (to borrow a term from Spitz) with one's internal objects, phantoms in one's head so to speak. I also want to say that I don't agree with Otto Kernberg about idealization. There is a difference between pushing other people into achieving what one wants to achieve oneself (consciously or unconsciously) and simply idealizing them.

Alejandro Tarnopolsky (U.K.).   I was very impressed with Dr. Kernberg's paper and want only to address a minor point which has to do with terminology. Could we not make use of the distinction, which Dr. Kernberg referred to briefly, between projecting onto and projecting into? This has, of course, to do with the distinction between placing something on the surface, or placing it inside. What I want to develop is the notion that perhaps this can be used to clarify the issue raised today of the different intensity of the projective processes, ranging from minimal to massive. One of the instruments of measurement of the projection is the analyst himself in his response to the dynamic field created between patient and analyst. This is not the only measure of the intensity, but it can be used to distinguish between those states where we can work with a tolerable state of comfort-discomfort, doubt, and the possibilities of gratification or interpretation of the patient's material. These are states in which we can observe what the patient makes us feel and deal more or less comfortably with it. They can be regarded as indicating some kind of projection that remains in some way peripheral or on the surface of our capacity to think, and I would like to suggest that these processes of projection of a lower intensity should be referred to as projections onto. All of these can be distinguished from the more intense processes where we are actually thrown off balance, which applies to all the many clinical examples given by both Miss Joseph and Dr. Kernberg. These involve processes where we lose command, get confused, are flooded with fantasies which we feel are not our own. The notion of varieties of countertransference described by Grinberg and Racker is implicit in what I am saying. I want to suggest that these processes should be referred to as those where the projection takes place into the analyst, as though the sting of the projection has penetrated beneath the skin. I should like to suggest that perhaps we can use this distinction offered by the English language to increase our precision.

Roni Solan (Israel). I am thankful to Dr. Kernberg for allowing me to get closer to the concept of projective identification, and should like to say that I am intrigued by the relation of projective identification to the integration of the patient's narcissistic state. I am thinking particularly of the third patient, who introjected his father but who felt that you were not a reliable person for him. How did this tie in with his narcissism? Could you comment on the sequence of the merging through projective identification and the subsequent threat to narcissistic integrity?

Abraham Braun (West Germany). Dr. Kernberg, your books have been extremely good transitional objects for me when I didn't know you. I want to comment that in the many patients I have seen who have been fatherless for a long time, transitional objects were not the good objects provided by the mother. Rather, the child, in his loneliness, introjected objects of his own choice, including aspects of his surroundings. I have had the opportunity during the analysis of these patients to see how these transitional objects can be given back, in a sense as a sort of gift from our patients. This can lead to the development of the transference neurosis proper.

Wolfgang Berner (Austria). I should like to ask Dr. Kernberg what the role of the father is in the development of projective identification?

M. Shoshani (Israel). I want to thank Dr. Kernberg for his beautiful presentation, although I find myself in disagreement with a number of points. Could you clarify why you regard projective identification as an earlier, more archaic mechanism than projection? Working with chronic schizophrenic patients I find that both mechanisms are prevalent. I think that in fact projection occurs more frequently, and if we accept the rule that the sicker the patient is, the more archaic the mechanisms he uses, then this would suggest that projection is the more primitive mechanism.

I also find myself in disagreement over the differentiation of borderline personality organization from schizophrenia; I have not found that an interpretation of projection or projective identification can differentiate the two. Finally, I think there is some contradiction between the concepts of holding and containment and the concept of systematic dissolution of the grandiose self. So in the first case you presented, the lady who felt that you were from a small town, I find that you did not adhere to the procedure of containment and holding, but that you went straight on with systematic dissolution of the grandiose self. I should like to hear your comments on this.

E. Oosterhuis (The Netherlands).   I want to ask a practical question about technique because you said, Dr. Kernberg, that what you did was debatable when you expressed your fear with your third patient. Most of my experience has been with children, and what you have said about your own work with disturbed patients reminds me of working with very disturbed children. With these children one often has to set limits and make them feel secure in order to work with them. Is it not also necessary to do this when you work with such disturbed adults? You could then feel safe without having to say to the patient that you were afraid. I have some doubts about the wisdom of expressing your fears to such patients, because in my experience with children this arouses guilt and may make them more fearful. One has to be very secure, I think, to provide a situation of safety for the patient, as if one were a holding mother. So I should like to ask whether there is a parameter of technique possible here in that one might change the setting when working with very aggressive patients. Perhaps one might have to work in a clinic where there are other people around who can come in to set limits, or some similar method.

Otto Kernberg.   I have been asked a number of very good questions, and I certainly will not be able to do justice to all of them. I shall try to pick those that I find easier to respond to; some of the questions raised would require that I spend much more time thinking them through.

I agree with Dr. Tarnopolsky that one might say that in the case of projection it is "onto" and projective identification "into." I find that convincing. In this connection Dr. Shoshani raised the question of why I believe that projective identification is earlier than projection, and he mentioned that he had seen both in schizophrenic patients. As I mentioned in my paper, in practically all the cases where I had originally thought that the schizophrenic patients were projecting, it turned out that they were making use of projective identification. I reached the conclusion, on an empirical clinical basis, that with neurotic (that is, healthier) patients one often finds them attributing properties to the analyst that the analyst doesn't possess, and to which he doesn't react particularly. One can absorb this into the transference while maintaining empathy with what is projected by the patient. Very often the projections are of issues about which the patient has no conscious awareness, nor has he the need to exert omnipotent control. In my view there is an early organization of defensive operations based upon splitting that predates the predominance of repression. I see projection as the projection of something that has been repressed. It is therefore a consequence of the mechanism of repression having taken over as a main organizing defensive operation. When Freud described projection he really described a set of very complex mechanisms, including what occurred in schizophrenic patients, and including as well what he considered was transformation of love into hatred. We think very differently about this issue now: it is not a transformation of love into hatred, but a splitting of love from hatred which is then very often dealt with through projective identification.

This brings me to the question raised by Dr. Braun regarding transitional objects. If I understand him correctly, it is not simply that in fatherless children a good father is missed, and a transitional object set up, but that the lack of a good parent activates a deep sense of frustration. To analyze such a situation further means that we have to analyze the complex internal situations that are precipitated or evoked by what seems to be, from the viewpoint of external reality, simply the absence of an object.

Now I would like to go to my third clinical case. I want to say first that of course I had to simplify the presentation of all the cases enormously. I wanted to give you sufficient information so that it could be seen how severely ill they were, and then I had to limit myself to microscopic episodes to show the mechanism of projective identification, singled out where possible. The price that one pays for this is that of losing a sense of the analytic process over an extended period of time. The advantage is, I hope, that it permits us to single out a particular psychological operation. My third patient had a combination of narcissistic and paranoid features in his personality, with a pathological grandiose self. At the same time, there was an infiltration of that self with aggression and there was abundant use of projective mechanisms to deal with this. In the relationship with me, the transference related to his father emerged as the first transference issue, and I took it up simply because that was what presented itself in the relation to me. It showed in the form of the two mutually split transferences I mentioned. These were an idealizing one connected with homosexual submission to such an ideal father, and a persecutory one. There was an endlessly repetitive activation of these, with the patient being stuck, so to speak, in the self aspect of the relationship. Now what is interesting is that the ideal good father was really unavailable to him except as a longed-for homosexual object that he couldn't tolerate. Love meant homosexual submission, and at this point in his analysis he couldn't identify with the sadistic father that was one aspect of his pathological grandiose self. I think what happened is that as we went along analyzing the split between these contradictory relations to his father the patient first became less afraid of his aggression because he realized that there was both love and hatred in him. So his tolerance of aggression increased, and now he became able at one point to activate in the transference, by means of the mechanism of projective identification, the sadistic aspects of his relationship with his father, with an inverse or reciprocal distribution of roles which before he was incapable of. For the first time I became his frightened self, and he became his sadistic father. I think the regressive aspects of this development may also be interpreted as a temporary dissolution of the pathological grandiose self, the patient being confronted with his primitive world of object relations, against which the grandiose self is a protection. Therefore the motive for identifying himself with the sadistic father was to maintain security under conditions of extreme danger. He had to face his aggression without the usual protection of the grandiose self and, by daring to identify with his own aggression, without having to project the sadistic father. At the same time he had to force me to submit to him and to help him maintain the rationalization for his rage: I had lied to him. So my "lying" was a precondition for the ego-syntonicity of his aggression, a defense against guilt and concern. I could not handle it, and this brings me to the question about the fear. Do I think one should confess one's emotions to the patient? Definitely not. I try to use my affective reactions as part of my interpretive comments. At that particular point with this patient I found myself in an extreme situation in which I felt that in reality I was about to be attacked. I felt that was a realistic fear. The patient was a tall, powerful man with a history of physical violence, and he had the intensity and the attitude that made me think there was a real danger there. I have worked with psychotic patients a great deal, so I don't think I was fearful or frightened beyond what was appropriate to the situation, but I was afraid to the extent that my work was interfered with. I felt therefore that I had to introduce what may be called a parameter of technique, a structuring of the situation, which meant moving out of the position of technical neutrality; and that is what I did. This was an effort to prevent the situation in which an act of violence might occur, one which I think would have provided further problems for the patient. I preferred to deal with it technically as I did, and I gave this example because it illustrates both the problems that were aroused in me and the use of the technique of facing patients with "incompatible realities." I might do this in other cases without expressing my own reaction.

Responding now to Mrs. Oosterhuis, I would say that there is a danger that talking about one's own anxieties may increase guilt in the patient. If I have moved away from a position of technical neutrality what I do is to interpret to the patient the reason that made me move away, and I try to reconstitute a position of neutrality by interpretive means. This may sometimes take weeks, but I think that it is possible to maintain an analytic situation in these circumstances. In answer to Dr. Solan, certainly the patient's narcissistic integrity was challenged or threatened, but it had a pathological narcissistic quality. We have to differentiate normal infantile narcissism from pathological narcissism, which needs to be analyzed so that more normal infantile narcissism can come to the fore. I think that was the case in my patient.

Dr. Shoshani's point that there is a contradiction between holding and containment as opposed to systematic dissolution of a pathological grandiose self is a good one. I hadn't thought of this before: it could be seen as a contradiction. My first reaction (although I must think about this further) is that the analysis of the pathological grandiose self is a long-term process. Containment or holding are short-term processes in which the analyst deals with what the patient cannot tolerate at that moment, with what he projects. The analyst then tries to control it himself. Containment and holding can then be understood in the sense of neither crumbling under the patient's aggression nor retaliating, but rather tolerating and transforming it into an interpretation. This is what we might call a tactical approach, whereas the systematic analysis of the transference might be seen as a strategic one.

Chapter 9

Projection, Identification, and Projective Identification: Their Relation to Political Process

RAFAEL MOSES

While projection and identification are psychological defense mechanisms with which all of us are by now well acquainted—even though we may differ about their definition or about how frequently they are used or found—projective identification is, as you will have gathered, a different kettle of fish. This is so because some of us have been nurtured on projective identification, so to speak, with our psychoanalytic mother's milk, whereas others among us have not. This creates a situation where those of us who have imbibed projective identification from early on tend to see this mechanism as ubiquitous and therefore highly important, and consequently believe that those who do not appreciate its importance lack a dimension of knowledge and a skill which add greatly to the capabilities of the analyst. They are therefore seen as greatly limited in the scope of their analytic work. On the other side are those who tend to hold to the opposite belief, namely, that projective identification perhaps does not exist at all as a special mechanism, or else is immensely overrated in its importance. The fuss made about it is regarded as blinding us to other phenomena, and perhaps as distorting the patient's material. When talking to analysts in different parts of the world, we can hear both these views expressed. Certainly we have all heard a lot about this mechanism in these past few days.

To hold strong beliefs in such a fashion is probably not consistent with the scientific attitude which some of us deem necessary in our profession. But interestingly, the very fact that such black-and-white beliefs are held with so much conviction brings us promptly into the other area with which I want to try to connect these mechanisms today, namely, the area of political process. There are similarities between the way strong beliefs are held in our professional circles and what we can observe in the wider political arena. In the domain of political process it is taken as the rule that people hold strong beliefs and convictions, and moreover are certain that what they believe in is right, while what the other believes is totally wrong. Thus we Israelis are convinced, by and large, that we are surrounded by nations who threaten our very existence; that it is the other side—the PLO, the Shiites, Jordan, Syria, or even the Palestinians in the West Bank and the Gaza strip (also called Judaea and Samaria)— which wishes to attack us, that they are callous and unconscionable, aggressive and not defensive in their posture. The other side, in its turn—strange as it may seem to most of us Israelis—holds the same belief about us. This phenomenon is sometimes called the "demonization" of the enemy and is well known not only in daily international or sectarian conflicts the world over, but also in scientific descriptions of such conflicts (Volkan, 1979; Moses, 1983a; 1983b). Does this mean that political process enters into our professional life? I am convinced that it does so, in a variety of ways, some of which I will return to later. But I would also like to say that psychological statements about political process need to be made in a much more tentative way than those we make about individuals. If we move now from our professional or psychoanalytic politics to consider the psychological aspects of political process, it is clear that such aspects will be discernible wherever political process exists, i.e., wherever there are emotional reactions in and between groups of human beings. The more strongly people feel, the more emotionally will political processes be affected. Perhaps I should say: the more *irrationally* will political process be affected. Since large groups in particular tend to elicit irrational rather than task-oriented reactions (see Bion, 1961), it will not surprise us to find this also in political process. And if we return now once more to political process in *our* professional, public, and private lives, it is my impression that projective identification is one of those concepts in psychoanalysis which elicits similar, not always rational reactions in many of us.

I would like to make another comment before I begin to consider our three mechanisms in more detail. It has to do with my position in this symposium. Looking around me, I perceive three distinguished participants, my colleagues who preceded me, of whom three or perhaps two (I am not sure about your psychoanalytic antecedents, Dr. Meissner!), did, so it seems to me, imbibe projective identification with their mother's milk. In addition I see our chairman, who grew up with one foot in such an environment. This leaves me in a somewhat isolated position, I feel. And let me comment that for a small group (in this case a group of one!) to find itself so isolated is a well-known situation in political process. This has certain psychological implications and consequences—of which it is useful to be aware, both for the person concerned, here for me, and for those around him, namely for all of you. Thus a person who feels isolated will inevitably feel more insecure. As a result he may respond in one or another of a variety of well-known ways: he may try to cover up what he sees as his vulnerability by defensive actions such as denial, arrogance, or aggressive behavior. On the other hand, the majority group in the panel this afternoon, those to whom the concept of projective identification comes naturally, may well have its own particular responses to the situation. And this is also true for the third partner, the onlookers, the audience i.e., most of you. The audience may identify with the majority or with the minority, depending on many factors, not the least of which is their feeling response to such a situation of conflict. This, then, is a further example of how both political process and its psychological correlates are conspicuous in human groups, including this group here today.

Allow me now to begin at the beginning. I would like to start with projection, which we all know. It is generally known that projection was first regarded as being mainly a psychotic mechanism. Freud's first published reference to projection deals with the distrust of other people becoming a replacement for self-reproach in the condition of paranoia (Freud, 1896, p. 184). It is of interest, I think, that the cumbersome but much oversimplified formulation of homosexual love turning into paranoia demonstrates a facet which brings it closer to projective identification, namely, that there is a continued connection between the person who projects and what has been projected into the other. In a study carried out some years ago (Moses and Halevi, 1972), a colleague and I differentiated between what we called partial and full projections. While the partial projection ascribed the projected material to the other person, it was *not* seen as being turned back toward the projector. In the full projection, however, that particular link with the object and with the material projected onto him is maintained—for example, when the object is now feared as a source of aggression. This full, more prevalent form of projection *does* show continued contact with the object, but this contact is not sufficient, in my view, to warrant our designating the process as projective identification.

So while originally the emphasis was on projection as a paranoid mechanism found mostly in very disturbed persons, we have all, I think, been able to convince ourselves from our therapeutic work, as well as from simply living in this world, that projection is a much more widely used mechanism than was originally thought. But I do not think that we have as yet done justice to the complexity of projection or the other mechanisms being considered. We see our patients project onto us their aggressive wishes and at times their sexual wishes. And we cannot fail to observe the projection of their superego onto us when they appoint us as their substitute consciences, or when they project their ego ideal onto us, a process which is involved in some forms of idealization.

Certainly we do not find it difficult to observe the workings of projective mechanisms in everyday life. We tend to blame others, not always quite rationally: the grocer who we think may have cheated us, the bureaucrat who, by procrastinating, seems to vent his bile on us, the taxi driver who took us the long way around and overcharged us. All such people will, of course, seem to want to "do us in," all the more when we are in alien territory, as many of you are at this moment, and as many of us are when we attend meetings abroad. One might wonder whether the operation of projection in this type of frequently encountered situation does not serve the discharge of amounts of aggression as it accumulates.

It is particularly easy to observe projection in certain group situations. One example is the army, a rigidly structured organization which does not allow for much direct expression of negative feelings. Thus it is often the sergeant-major upon whom aggressive tendencies and wishes are projected, so that he is seen as a threatening, bullying, and in general feared and hated figure. This projection occurs presumably because of the structure of the army and the psychological implications of this structure, and also because the function and behavior of the sergeant-major so easily lend themselves to his being the bearer of aggression, and to being viewed as such. Yet here another question may be raised. Some of you may feel that the everyday projective mechanisms with which we are all familiar are different in quality from the more openly paranoid trends which we see mainly in psychotics. Is the same basic mechanism operating in both? Is it only a question of degree, or of strength of projection—where perhaps quantity at some point determines quality? Or should we focus on how much of our sense of reality we retain?

There is another social area, quite familiar to us, where the projection of aggressive tendencies can be observed. I mean, of course, our professional societies and institutions. In these, where emotionally intense relationships exist among people who care about what they do—and therefore argue and fight about it—political processes necessarily take place. Thus we often find a member—could it at times be ourselves?—regarding another member as "the villain." We will hope that it is not ourselves who are thus regarded. He who finds himself viewed as the villain will often in turn see his antagonist very similarly. And as each thus views the other, he finds his own self-image enhanced by having an archenemy. In this way the projection of hostility and the creation of an enemy—in organizational as in other politics—provides two narcissistic benefits. We are as good as the "others" are bad; and our importance increases because we have archenemies. This view of political process in our professional and organizational institutions yields a picture which I think is not unfamiliar to most of us.

Let us now leave both projection and our societies and institutions, and look at the next defense mechanism on our list today: identification. This mechanism has been much more easily recognized and widely accepted than projective identification, and also more than projection. We are all familiar with identification as it occurs in various stages of development, in particular in its role as an intrinsic part of object relationships. We identify with those we love and are close to, and we make use of identification to help us deal with separations from our love objects. In the process, identification serves the function of structure building, so essential for development. Generally our identifications are more visible to the outsider than to ourselves. They become more evident when they operate after we have mourned the loss of someone we have loved.

Identification can help to demonstrate a useful distinction with regard to the duration of a defense mechanism over time. As in the examples I have given, identification is usually considered as operating over the long term. Yet a shorter, more transitional form of identification takes place quickly, and therefore much more often, in our daily interactions with others. Some years ago Joseph Sandler talked to me about how, when we see a stranger faltering a few meters from us, we feel, somehow, somewhere, in relation to our own body the "almost falling" of the other (Sandler and Joffe, 1967). Our ego boundaries will be momentarily inattentive and allow us to identify briefly with the stranger in this "almost falling." We will therefore try to counteract the hardly noticeable, momentarily unpleasant sensation. We do so either by the fantasy, acted out in a minute way, of righting our body so as not to fall; or by disidentifying with the person who stumbles. Both mechanisms serve our need to be reassured that what happens to the other does not happen to us, that we are different from him. Some years ago I applied this view to the soldier in battle (Moses, 1978) and asked, Must he not identify—fleetingly, perhaps for a part of a second—with the enemy at whom he aims his weapon, particularly if he can actually see him as a living person? And then must he not as quickly disidentify, in order to be able to aim to kill? Similarly, he will identify more basically with the aggression of the enemy, with a transitoriness which will depend on the circumstances of the specific battle, or on the morale of his unit and his society and on his basic personality. This will allow him to be the aggressor he needs to be, to do what needs to be done for his country, and no less to protect his own life. This sort of almost-reflex identification with the aggressor enters into the two different chronological forms of identification. On the one hand, it reinforces the more stable and continuous, partly conscious identification which plays a part in maintaining his identity as a fighting soldier. On the other hand, the transitory unconscious identification is suddenly strengthened as he observes aggressive acts around him. Thus he will find himself, willy-nilly, being like the friend or foe who commits acts seen as inhuman, yet which are also felt to be inescapably necessary in order to survive (see Moses, 1978). The concept of dehumanization is clearly related to this phenomenon. I refer here to how people are brought to view members of another group as less than human. In the dehumanizing process, identifications with the enemy, even transient ones, act as interferences and have to be counteracted.

A soldier who became a psychological casualty after participating in battle recalled a frightening image only after a fair amount of therapeutic working through of his acute anxiety state. He visualized seeing through the sight of his gun a young, blond boy—not even a man—who looked very much like him or like one of his friends. Such a recollection leads us to ask whether he had become a casualty precisely because he was unable to totally repress this temporary identification, this transient feeling of oneness with the enemy.

Such transitory identifications occur in us wherever we are: in an audience listening to the speaker, as you are doing now; as a speaker speaking to an audience as I am doing; at a professional conference where we meet colleagues from other countries with whom we share experiences. But we have come to know such transitory identifications most often and with most awareness through our experience of the psychoanalytic hour. Here we can examine them most directly, particularly in ourselves as therapists. Isn't this what we do day in, day out, hour after hour when we listen to the patient, when we follow his thoughts, words, and feelings? While we do so we maintain a stable long-term identification with the patient. At the same time we find that the emotional distance between us

varies and fluctuates. From listening with empathy and a floating attention that requires a certain distance, ready to hearken to our inner
thoughts and feelings, we move at times to a deeper and stronger identification with the patient. Then the emotional distance has become short-
ened. Relatively soon, we move back to a more observing stance, toward
both the other and ourselves, for which we need a greater distance. At
times we test how "in tune" we are with our patient by seeing whether we
can predict his trend of thought, or even the next words he will utter.
Often our predictions are correct. Such a stance is an example of a greater
degree of identification coming into play for a short period within the
hour.

    It seems to me that there are different degrees as well as different
kinds of identification which we weave in and out of during an analytic
hour. But different degrees and different types of identification can also be
observed to exist in more stable ways during different stages of a treatment. We have not focused enough on these phenomena and on the
process of identification inherent in them, on the ways in which this
process varies, and how these variations are related to emotional distance.
What facilitates increased identification at a given point in time? What
makes us, at another time, pull back more? Which degrees and which types
of identification by the therapist are beneficial for the therapeutic process?
Which should serve us as warning signals? Only once we have understood
more about this area will we be able to apply our knowledge to groups and
therefore in turn to political process.

    What we can observe, however, are identifications occurring, for
example, in the negotiating representatives of two opposing groups—be
they industrialists and labor, antagonistic nations, or any other social
groups in conflict. The delegates of each group inevitably identify with the
representatives of the antagonists—of the other side—during negotiations (Jaques, 1955). This mutual identification allows representatives to
move more easily toward agreement with the other side than can the
people they represent, who have been left behind and have not been
directly involved in the negotiations. But it is because these identifications
are not shared by those at home that representatives have such difficulty
in convincing those they represent—including their leaders—to accept
the compromises they have made. An example of a much more short-lived
identification in political process is that made by millions of people with
Neil Armstrong, the astronaut who was the first man to step on the moon.
He invited people to identify with him when he said, "That's one small
step for a man but one giant leap for mankind!" I think this example also

illustrates some of the narcissistic gains that can result from such identifications—not only identifications with the first man to step on the moon, but also with the acts or statements of leaders. Some leaders invite their followers to share in the greatness offered to the large group. Churchill in Britain's most difficult hours in World War II comes to mind, but we can also think of demagogic leaders who tempt their followers with promises they cannot keep. And we have known for a long time that the more stable and long-term identifications of followers with their leaders, and with the goals and causes they represent, also provide narcissistic supplies (see Freud, 1921). Of course, identifications with the other members of the group are another hallmark of such group membership (Freud, 1921).

If identification can be viewed as constantly occurring, appearing and disappearing, waxing and waning as we continually relate to those around us, this should hold equally for other defense mechanisms. They must have the same transient as well as long-term patterns of operation. This would certainly hold true for projection, which clearly takes place on a stable, consistent, long-term basis. We see this, for example, in the projective viewing of a demonized enemy as the embodiment of all the evil we do not wish to see in ourselves. But projection can also be seen to appear and disappear, to strengthen and weaken from moment to moment, in our daily patterns of relating. As we deal in our daily encounters with our wives and husbands, with our children and our parents, our friends and our enemies, we constantly ascribe to them some of our own unconscious wishes and split-off affects, our proscriptions and our aspirations. As we project, just as when we identify, we sometimes move closer to our loved or hated ones, and at times a little further away from them.

In political behavior we will see many examples of such projections. Brief projections appear as we listen to the election speeches of candidates with whom we disagree. A transient superego projection can also be seen in the expectation of punishment by the enemy for an aggressive action carried out. It similarly occurs in the expectation of being found out for a transgression not yet discovered. Medium-term projection shows up in our view of enemies or scapegoats within our society who evoke projective proclivities for a limited period of time. German Jews in Palestine were thus targets for a number of years for the projection of qualities thought to be peculiar to them (being pedantic or slow on the uptake) until they were shunted aside for the next ethnic group to become the focus for the projection of different qualities. Public attitudes toward the territories occupied by Israel, which have not been assimilated—psychologically, politically, or legally—reflect more than just transient superego projections in Israel. But stable, consistent projection is perhaps most clearly seen in the hostility toward a long-term enemy—the surrounding Arab nations for us Israelis and vice versa. We can say the same for the Soviets and the Americans, and at one time for the Germans and the French. All these have made much use of the demonization of the enemy. But demonization is found equally *within* a society, vis-à-vis other groups polarized against one's own, be they ethnic, political, or religious in nature. An unusual and remarkable example of what seems to have been a massive projection of primitive material involving id and superego, as well as ego functions, could be observed in relation to the Reverend Jim Jones and his People's Temple in Jonestown, Guyana, which led to the mass suicide of the entire group. Much might be learned from a more detailed study of what happened there (Mills, 1979).

Projections of the ego ideal can be discerned in projections onto leaders anywhere—as was the case in Jonestown. But I suggest that such projections might usefully be divided into two kinds: projection of idealized qualities and projection of the judging function that determines what qualities are to be idealized. In political process the projection of idealized qualities is most noticeable when people delegate their striving for ideal goals to their leaders and to the group. Jim Jones's community seemed to be built on such behavior, when people were willing to serve blindly the needs of the leader and the group as he defined them. But perhaps ego ideal projection is equally involved when we look at our political enemies. What we find striking in our enemies is the absence of idealized qualities. Projection of the function that judges what is ideal and what is not is manifested more subtly in political process. It can become evident in a severe judging function, delegated to one's leaders, for which a highly moral person such as Ben Gurion provided a most suitable vehicle for us Israelis. Having a leader of this sort, many felt that they could safely relinquish to him such judging functions, and accepted his judgment blindly. They, or we, thereby avoided the burden of responsibility for decisions based on such judging functions. Such abdication of personal responsibility has been described by many as part of group membership (LeBon, 1920; Freud, 1921; Scheidlinger, 1952). Interestingly, projection of the judging function is equally involved when following a leader who shows a *lack* of moral scruples, who subverts ideals. He too is followed blindly, again because a leader has become the sole carrier of judging functions. Examples range from Sharon here in Israel to Nixon in the

United States—and probably, in a more extreme form, to Jim Jones in Jonestown.

At times what is projected can be extremely primitive or inconsistent. We see this in the projection of the archaic, primitive superego of delinquents or criminals who show superego lacunae. When projected onto others, such superego content remains archaic, punitive, and inconsistent. This is also true for so-called corruptible superegos, as shown by Richard Nixon—president and leader of his people—in what is now known as the Watergate Affair (Rangell, 1980). Two interesting tidbits which show how Nixon perceived others and what they did to him or to his friends have recently become public knowledge and point up the primitive and immature aspects of the superego as well as its projection. When asked whether he had approved the effort to have the head of the CIA interrupt the investigation of the Watergate affair by the FBI, Nixon recently replied, "Of course I approved it—we had done enough for him, so why shouldn't he do something for us now?" Nixon also related that when he learned that two of his friends were in trouble with the income tax authorities, he became furious and immediately issued an order that since the income tax people were harassing his friends, they should do the same to his enemies, the Democratic leaders (*Newsweek*, April 16, 1984). Perhaps the readiness to project superego and ego ideal qualities also determines why some leaders—and their followers—are more likely than others to espouse ideals and ideologies, particularly stringent all-or-nothing ones. These instill in their movement the readiness to fight Holy Wars—figuratively or literally. The lofty end will then justify all means. Examples in political process are legion; they range from the relatively moderate adherence to a stringent ideology in the pre-State population of Israel, through the Watergate Affair, to Khomeinism and Shiite religiously based suicide missions.

Let me now proceed to our third mechanism, which includes the first two but has a quality and function uniquely its own. This is the one, I need not remind you, which for many is the most difficult to comprehend and the hardest to accept. I personally have particular difficulty with what has been posited as the basis for the institution of projective identification (Klein, 1931, 1946), i.e., the death instinct. I belong to the large group of analysts who consider the death instinct theory to be a none-too-convincing speculation by Freud (1937, 1940); the majority of analysts today do not accept it. In any event, I remain unable to fathom why the death instinct would need to be seen as a prerequisite for the understanding of projective identification.

To look at the mechanism, let me turn to a clinical example. A thirty-year old woman, one and a half years in analysis, had as one of her main concerns a fear that people close to her "would die on her." On occasion she would laugh and talk in a lighthearted way, while the content of her thoughts related to somber matters or even to acts of cruelty. The analyst gradually became aware of a feeling of sadness in herself, the source of which she could not immediately identify. Following a remark by the patient that the analyst looked unhappy and that she, the patient, wished that she could do something about this, the analyst could interpret that the patient seemed to push her sadness away from herself and over to the analyst. In the next session the patient reported a dream of the night before in which she cried. Her associations led to a memory from age nine relating to the sudden death of her grandmother. She cried bitterly during this hour, and thus in a sense retrieved the sadness she had pushed out of herself. Many of us would agree that such phenomena are not infrequent, and that they consist, in the first place, of a projection of affect—the unacknowledged sadness of the patient which "suddenly" appeared in the analyst, as if from nowhere. But can we see here an identification with what has been projected?

Before I answer that question, let me move to the third requirement for projective identification, namely, the influence or control exerted, in fantasy or reality, over what has been projected and is identified with and over the love object who is the carrier of what has been projected. It must be clear that when we speak of control in this context we mean something much more than the control exerted over our wishes or impulses by simply using one or the other defense mechanism or defensive maneuver. In the patient I have just described, the attempt to control, relevant to projective identification, was evidenced in her concern about the analyst's unhappiness, and in her wish to help. She could not help herself with her split-off sad feelings, but she attempted to do so once she had located them in the analyst.

Those among us who have difficulty accepting the ubiquity of the mechanism of projective identification can nevertheless often locate it quite easily in psychotic patients. In fact, many descriptions of the mechanism use examples drawn from such patients (e.g., Thorner, 1955). Perhaps early psychotherapists related to more disturbed patients in a way that made it possible to identify mechanisms in them which could not be discerned in the neurotic patients because these had a closer resemblance to their therapists. Only in the last two or three decades has it become more generally accepted that many of the mechanisms previously described for psychotic patients (perhaps all of them) are ubiquitous. They are to be found not only in all our patients, but in ourselves. (And of course, they abound in our colleagues!)

Let us now see if we can observe projective identification in groups, which represent a step on the way from the individual to political process. In a class of twelve-year-olds, one youngster suddenly erupted against the teacher. While the others were not moved in this case to join in (see Redl, 1966, on the subject of contagion in groups), it was not difficult to learn that at that moment they shared anger at the teacher. In a situation that did not easily permit such an expression of anger, one group member could express it with unconscious covert support from the others, who shared vicariously the relief of having pent-up angry feelings expressed, even if not by direct action of their own. They shared the gratification of seeing the teacher under attack. We can understand, then, that the youngsters in some way projected their anger into one of their group, someone who had been selected and who had unconsciously offered himself for selection in those half-understood ways in which families select their scapegoats (see Vogel and Bell, 1960). The sudden projection of anger at a crucial point in time afforded the group members the opportunity to control a split-off affect that was now external to them. By affecting the behavior of one of their members, they affected the classroom situation and the teacher. The spokesman for the anger of the whole class was certain to be punished. Through this, the members of the class could feel that their own "illegitimate" anger was under control, but that they could at the same time escape the pain of retribution. They could also experience some narcissistic gain through being at one with the teacher. We can thus see here the three cardinal signs of projective identification and the wish to exert control over what has been projected.

The identification that follows the projection of affects or wishes is particularly evident when the group member onto whom they are projected is—or becomes—a group leader. In these group instances, the wish of the group members for continued contact with the projected content is evident and convincing in a variety of ways, because the continuing identification is so evident.

An analyst began a therapeutic group for some patients who were at the same time in individual psychotherapy or analysis with her. A surprising element in the group's behavior was soon noted. A young man had—in individual treatment—consistently behaved in a polite, friendly, and sometimes very warm way toward his analyst, while providing indirect indications of hostility. His behavior changed markedly quite soon after joining the group. He seated himself opposite the therapist in the circle and berated her in ways for which he sought to enlist group support. This hostile, aggressive trait had not come out openly in his analysis. It was only now, as he found himself more distant from his analyst, in physical terms as well as emotionally and socially, that he acted otherwise than in the one-to-one situation. One aspect of his personality, his partially split-off aggressive feelings toward the analyst, had previously been less available for direct scrutiny. In the group these feelings received unconscious support from the group members and from the group climate. The group members chose him to be the spokesman of group aggression toward the therapist. Viewed from the other side, we could say that they accepted his *offer* to be such a spokesman. This changed state of affairs now enabled him to make contact with and to express his previously split-off aggressiveness. This patient with the support of the other group members—or the group members with his help—could now exercise control over their aggressive feelings in a different way.

Clearly, politicians frequently serve as the target for the projection of a variety of wishes and affects which the projector cannot directly express or even consciously tolerate within himself. Leaders, as we have seen, are also the recipients of projected superego material. The expectation of being judged and perhaps punished for wishes and affects known only to ourselves manifests itself most easily in our fear of being found out by the official representatives of our leaders and of society: most frequently it is policemen whom we see or imagine. Followers also delegate to their leaders the authority to judge what is right and what is wrong, what is admirable and to be strived for, and what is not. Those among us who have difficulty in identifying with our national leaders find it much easier to project our *unacceptable* feelings and wishes upon them (unfortunately a widespread Israeli experience these days).

If we look for instances in political process which show the wish to exert control in addition to projection and identification, other examples come to mind. We might say that the members of Gush Emunim, that ultranationalistic group of settlers in territories on the other side of what we call the green line (the 1967 boundaries of Israel), projectively identified with the one-time Prime Minister Menachem Begin. This was more than simple identification because they also thereby pushed him to adopt some of their extreme positions. Viewing it from the other side, we might say that Mr. Begin projectively identified with the extreme position of Gush Emunim, which could enact some of the views that he could not allow himself to express directly. By egging them on—probably unconsciously—to maintain a consistently— more militant position, he in fact served his own ends in several ways. Probably quite intentionally, as well as unconsciously, he covered his right flank politically. But he was also enabled to maintain a less extreme position. This is analogous to the parent who can rely on the other parent to consistently maintain an extreme position—being, for example, the stern one in bringing up the children, or the one who is a "free spender." So we see in the dyad—the group of two—a process that often occurs in or between groups: namely, one protagonist is able to maintain a one-sided position precisely because he can be sure that the other will consistently represent the other side of the argument, i.e., of the ambivalence. In the example of Gush Emunim, Mr. Begin could use their extreme political position as leverage for being somewhat responsive—and yet not too responsive—to the constituency on his extreme right. Mr. Reagan in the United States is in a similar position now with his extreme right—from which he needs to take some distance without losing their support.

Here the mixture of conscious intent and less conscious motivation can be seen very well. They are difficult to keep apart, particularly, I believe, because they constantly coexist side by side. Thus Mr. Begin's covert invitation to extreme activism from the right wing of his coalition—an activism he could not let himself condone—provided him vicarious gratification for deeds he could not consciously approve. (Recent poignant events in Israel have made these comments particularly pertinent.) There is in this situation again an analogy to family psychodynamics. A parent will covertly encourage a child to act out wishes that are consciously unacceptable yet which provide vicarious gratification (see Ackerman, 1958; Wynne, 1965; Haley and Hoffman, 1967; and, with regard to the use of projective identification in the family, Zinner and Shapiro, 1972; Zinner, 1976).

We encounter here a sometimes quite confusing aspect of the relationship between unconscious processes and external reality. In this context it has been said that the person who feels inappropriately persecuted is nonetheless supported by an existing external reality—there is a grain of truth in his feelings of persecution. At the very least, it is the reality that his "enemy"—usually also his unconscious love object—does in fact harbor unconscious aggressive wishes against him (see Freud, 1922). Lidz (1965) has stated the interesting proposition that the megalomania of the schizophrenic has a basis in reality in the sense that he really is the centerpiece of the world—usually his mother's world. Henry Kissinger in a different context said that even someone who is paranoid can still be persecuted in reality.

We will always expect to see a consistent interaction between inner and outer reality in all psychic mechanisms. Indeed, the psychoanalytic conception of object relationships and unconscious processes makes such a connection inevitable. The important "other" and the environment are always directly or indirectly involved in all intrapsychic mechanisms. They have a constant impact upon the individual. Thus we say that the analysand who "caused" her analyst to feel unexpectedly sad must have brought to the fore some of the analyst's own sadness. This could occur only if some such sadness had existed within the analyst—latently, if you will. To phrase it differently, projection does not involve projecting psychic content into a vacuum. Rather we see a mechanism that stimulates, facilitates, or strengthens psychic content already there, a mechanism based on preexisting content in the receiver. We would usually expect to find a mixture of the two—a projection onto or into the other, together with the existence of psychic content in the receiver that serves as a basis on which the projection then builds and expands. It might be interesting to speculate about cultural differences in this respect.

These mixtures of fact and fantasy, of reality and idiosyncratic perception, build belief systems that deviate from reality in individuals and in groups, yet contain elements of reality. In large groups and in political process, these phenomena are often both striking and confusing. To return to the example of Gush Emunim, it seems beyond doubt that the members of this group intentionally and with much conscious effort attempted to influence the national leader to act in accordance with their activist views. They would do so both by arguing their case and by a variety of political maneuvers. But such real and intentional behavior by no means excludes the operation of concurrent unconscious mechanisms. Gush Emunim and the national leader also interact through mechanisms of unconscious egging on, and thus gain vicarious gratification, a mechanism well known to us from the studies of the psychodynamics of the family (Ackerman, 1958; Wynne, 1965; Haley and Hoffman, 1967). This mechanism of vicarious gratification—described by Ruth Eissler (1953) for what she called the scapegoats of society—is closely related to projective identification.

I should like to make it clear that I am not speaking here of consciously contrived activities. My point is that while we psychoanalysts and psychotherapists have become accustomed to viewing conscious and unconscious motivation as continuously existing side by side in the individual, we are not used to applying this view to the large group. In political process most people—including psychodynamically oriented professionals—are disproportionately aware of external reality, and accord less legitimacy (if any) to the concurrent existence of a constant flow of unconscious motivations. Such an attitude is understandable because large groups are not our patients. It is natural to be much more diffident in assuming the existence of unconscious processes where we do not perceive them daily, as we do in our work. My suggestion is that these two differently occurring and differently motivated ways of behaving—the conscious and the unconscious—need to be seen as existing side by side in the family, and in groups both large and small, no less than in the individual. This is demonstrable in political process. The affinity between Gush Emunim settlers and Mr. Begin made for both psychological and practical interactions. Emotional and unconscious motives existed inter-twined with practical and reality-based interactions. Of course, the unconscious basis of the relationship between leaders and followers is much less accessible to our view than is their seemingly rational behavior. And they are also less accessible to us than is the unconscious basis of behavior and of relating in the individuals who are our patients, be they leaders or followers. Our own reluctance to deal with this subject bases itself, in its rational aspect, on the fact that neither large groups nor most of the world's leaders come to us ready to expose themselves.

Some proponents of projective identification as a wide-ranging phe-nomenon describe an interesting interaction between the two members of the mother-child dyad. Ogden (1982), Grotstein (1982), and also Meissner (1980) view projective identification as an instrument which not only furthers the development of the child through its constant use but which requires or permits the other, the mother specifically, to help the devel-opment of the child. Thus they conceive of a constantly recurring process of projection and identification of psychic content felt to be "bad" or unacceptable to the infant. Such projective identification now allows the mother to modify the projected content and "hand it back" to the infant in a moderated, muted, and more acceptable way. This, of course, is Bion's view (1963) of the mother as a "container." Projective identification understood in this way then becomes specifically a psychic mechanism which can further the adaptive and integrative growth of the infant. This will happen when the good mother is able to accept and contain her child's unacceptable wishes and feelings. If the mother is unable to do so, the projected content will be returned in unmodified and therefore "bad" form, and will cause obvious difficulties. Implicit here is an analogy, not only to the analyst as a possible good mothering figure, but also to the leader and his function for the large group. The followers project content that is unacceptable to them onto (or into) their leader. Such content may be accepted by the leader in its raw and primitive form, by analogy to the projected material of the infant. It can thus be "returned" or reflected back to the leader's constituents in moderated and more acceptable form, less threatening and less raw and archaic. This would be the case with a moderate leader, the parallel to a good mother. Both are more at peace with themselves and with their own impulses and affects. The extreme, rigid leader, on the other hand, would not only be unable to moderate such projections but would perhaps even thrive on them. He would use them for escalating a conflictual situation, for polarization of attitudes and for demagogic dramatization. A warmer, more flexible, more moderate leader would make his constituents feel better about themselves by being a more tolerant and containing person, and would thereby encourage a more moderate, mature, flexible, and permissive social system. A tough, rigid leader would lead his followers to more extreme positions and to more aggressive behavior because of his psychological inability to tolerate or hold unacceptable psychic content in himself. The possible existence of such a mechanism in political process opens up fascinating possibilities.

This analogy from dyadic interrelations to political process has one other aspect. The analyst empathizes with the split-off unconscious aspects of his analysand's personality—with his wishes and affects—in an effort to understand the other person and to make unconscious, frightening material more acceptable to him. We can assume that a similar process takes place between the leader and his followers. But whereas the analyst makes a point of desisting from encouraging the blind translation of unconscious urges and fantasies into behavior, the leader and his followers will often tend to stimulate each other toward behavior that expresses conflicts directly through action rather than through thought. Here, too, there will be an opportunity for the leader to exercise a "bad" or a "good" mothering function toward his followers. He may empathize with and pick up those split-off parts of his followers which are more raw, unbridled, and archaic and, for example, through the use of demagoguery whip up a polarization of attitudes, extremism, and aggressive behavior. Alternatively, the good leader will empathize with and pick up or resonate to more mature and moderate psychic content. Or, if he tunes in to more primitive material, he will moderate it as he "returns" it to his constituents. The leader, depending on what sort of leadership pattern he establishes (analogous to mothering patterns), will either moderate or escalate the tensions within his followers. This has repercussions on the social group he leads and, finally, on the larger social system of which they—and other groups—form a part. (An example would be Muammar Kaddafi and his influence first on his followers, secondly on his society, and thirdly on the international conflicts of which he and his society are an integral part.)

By way of summary, I would like to suggest that the three mechanisms we have been discussing (including the most controversial one—projective identification) can help us clarify our thinking about groups as well as about individuals. This allows us to map out areas which require further study. We can pose new questions and perhaps look at familiar material from a different perspective.

The concept of projective identification, about which we have heard so much, also illustrates a point about concepts in general. A flexible definition of a concept allows us to use it adaptively and to modify it as necessary. Sandler (1983) has shown that we all tend to make use of concepts in much more idiosyncratic ways than we know or would like to think. In addition to the fertile, adaptive side of such unintentional ways of treating concepts, flexibility of this kind involves a serious danger. The overflexible use of the term projective identification by many authors (certainly by Grotstein, perhaps by Ogden and others) is detrimental because the widening of the term can cause it to lose its meaning. It is liable to become an undifferentiated catchall. Phenomena are then included which seem totally alien to the basic concept, as many would understand it. We must be beware, therefore, not only of too much rigidity in defining a term, but also of too much flexibility, lest the term lose its essential meaning.

Chapter 10

Discussion of Rafael Moses's Paper

Joseph Sandler. We have heard an extremely stimulating paper, one which may be rather disturbing for some of us. I think we have been shown how ubiquitous the mechanism of projective identification is. We tend to think that something which is irrational is abnormal, but of course this is not the case. Something can be both irrational and normal, and it seems clear that we have to regard the processes we have been discussing as part of the normal irrational interaction between the group we belong to and other groups. It leads one to think that there may be an important function for projective identification, both for the individual and the group. I am reminded here of the Jewish story, which I am sure many of you know, of the man who was shipwrecked, and lived for many years on his own on a desert island. He was a religious Jew who proceeded to do the best he could on the island, building himself a house and some other buildings. Finally a ship came along and saw the man's distress signal. An officer and some crew members arrived and wanted to take the shipwrecked man off. He was pleased about this, but asked them first to see what he had done. So he took them on a tour. He showed them his house and they were very impressed, and then he took them to a very fine hut he had constructed. He said, "This is my synagogue where I go to pray." They were equally impressed with this and then he said, "But I want to show you something else which is very important," and he took them to another building he had constructed and said, "And this is the synagogue I wouldn't set foot in if my life depended on it." It does seem that we need this sort of thing. I remember Anna Freud saying, on one of those occasions when she was being encouraged by some colleagues to withdraw from the British Psycho-Analytical Society, that she didn't think it was a good idea, because while we were in the British Society we remained a coherent group, and would certainly split into two or three groups if we separated from the other

151

analysts in the Society. I am sure that she was quite right about this. I think that a lot of what we call sadomasochistic behavior occurring between two people, or between groups, can be understood also as a provoking of the other to be the "bad" one, using the process of projective identification we have been discussing. If we can make the others bad we can be the good ones, just as Rafael Moses has described.

Lajos Székely (Sweden).   I was very impressed by the reference Dr. Moses made to those who were brought up on projective identification with their mother's milk. I was one of those who were not, who started internalizing the concept later, and had difficulties with it. I want to say a little about how projection is used in the political process, and how one selected the target for the projection of one's hostile impulses. In regard to Nazi propaganda during the second World War, a study has shown that the attribution of devilish characteristics to the Jews involved the attribution only of masculine characteristics, not feminine ones. The image of the Jew found in such propaganda goes back to the Shakespearean vision as depicted, for example, in Shylock. Literary analysis shows that in post-Shakespearean tradition it is always the male Jew who is disagreeable, while the Jewish woman appears as a pleasant, agreeable person. The question is, then, Why are only Jewish male characteristics projected, not female ones? I don't know, but I would like to pose the question.

How does the mechanism of projection operate? I think it is by means of a particular cognitive function, described by Imre Hermann, called selective thinking. The mechanism consists of selecting a small subgroup within a large group, the small group then becoming the representative of the total one. This could be seen, for example, in the Middle Ages, when court Jews were selected as representative of their people. This led to the idea that Jews were exploiters and usurers. This is an old tradition in the European myth, one that entered into the Nazi belief, and one that even Karl Marx accepted as part of his thinking about the Jews. Some court Jews were very influential and ambitious, and this provided the vehicle for the idea that Jews aspire to world domination.

J. Stelzer (Israel).   While I am from Israel, I was born in Buenos Aires and brought up with Kleinian concepts, which for many years were part of everyday life in psychotherapy, psychiatry, and psychoanalysis. Psychoanalytic concepts were also used freely to try to explain the political reality there. My past experience has impressed on me the possibility of the misuse of psychoanalytic concepts in this enterprise, and the dangers that this kind of approach might have. Let me illustrate this by mentioning my experience in the Argentine when I heard from my patients, from the political right and from the left as well, that there were concentration camps. When I told this to my colleagues they said, "Look, you are projecting." We used to comfort ourselves by saying that we were projecting. And we may be doing exactly the same in Israel nowadays because we want to achieve peace with our neighbors. So we may say that we project in order not to see that we are denying. To this we must add the fact that the political process influences the analytic situation, perhaps through projective identification, because our patients are very actively involved in political reality.

Finally, I do not think you have differentiated enough, Dr. Moses, between extremism and rigidity. I am not sure that extremism is always rigidity. For example, what would have happened to the Jews of this country if a group of people in 1948 had not been extremists?

Emanuel Berman (Israel). One of the most intriguing parts of this paper was the section on the possible political analogues of the positive uses of projective identification and the process of metabolizing them. However, I did find that part incomplete. Dr. Moses listed two types of leader, the extreme and the moderate. But if we go back to the therapeutic analogy, we can see three types of analyst. There is the analyst who is overtaken by the projection and therefore cannot metabolize it. There is the other extreme, the analyst who completely rejects the projective identification and therefore also cannot metabolize it. The patient cannot, as a result, experience that he has succeeded to any degree in the projective process. Finally there is the third type, who to some extent accepts the projection and then returns it in a modified way. This is the only one who is successful in achieving therapeutic change. Now if we follow this analogy, it has some interesting and innovative implications for the political process because it helps us understand the political failure of the ideological left, particularly in societies where intense nationalistic emotions are very prominent. What I am thinking of is the fate of those who are called "nigger-lovers" or, in this country, "Arab-lovers." If we take the Israeli scene, the left wing political leaders have failed in their attempts to change the popular, anti-Arab nationalistic sentiment because they are experienced by most people as being too foreign, too alien, and completely unaccepting of the projective identificatory needs for sharing in the extreme nationalistic emotion. It seems as if we experience these leaders as alien and moralistic, as assuming a superego function, as people who keep telling us that we are doing something wrong, that our feelings are illegitimate. As a result they are hated by a large segment of the population. The more successful effort to metabolize, to detoxify, the intense nationalistic emotions is that of the much less ideological, much less consistent, and perhaps less pleasant figures in the political world. So the politicians in this country who have a military background become acceptable figures for identification, and they are then in a position to be able to detoxify and return to the mass of the population the emotions projected onto them, now in a different form. One of the few examples in recent Israeli history of a successful metabolization of strong nationalistic sentiment can be seen in the relative acceptance of the Camp David accords.

Naomi Mibashan (Israel).   I want to say how much I was interested in the way Dr. Moses related projective identification to group and family processes, and to politics, particularly in Israel. As one of those for whom projective identification is good milk, I want to take up a small point in the paper with which I have some disagreement. I am not sure that there must always be, in the person who receives the projective identification, some psychic content or tendency that has to be complementary, that has to be the same as or similar to the psychic content being projected. I would rather stress what Leon Grinberg has said about projective counteridentification. This is a very special quality of countertransference in which we unconsciously react to the patient's transference, to his projective identification. This reaction is first unconscious, and then we try to deal with it, to make something out of it consciously. So what we perceive is the analyst's reaction to the massive projective identification of the patient. We can see reactions of anger, of boredom, of sadness, of confusion, and of similar emotions in working with groups of therapists in supervision. The story of a patient being treated by one of the therapists in such a group may produce a reaction in the entire group, which thereby receives the impact of the projective identification of a patient they don't even know. So I think we ought to take into account the analyst's reaction to the intensity of the projective identification of the patient, the analyst's projective counteridentification. This is not, of course, the same thing as countertransference.

Michael Conran (U.K.).   I want to say how much I appreciate Dr. Moses's having tackled a problem in a way that needed a great deal of courage. Projective identification has, of course, been with us a very long time. It is well recognized in Yiddish, and I am sure that Mrs. Klein would forgive me for drawing attention to an old saying that translates "He crawls around in your very bones." The English don't let people in so deep, so they say, "He gets under your skin."

Joseph Sandler.   Perhaps Dr. Conran can add to his collection of

Yiddish sayings another one pertinent to the discussion, namely, what in English would be "the capacity to talk oneself into having a cat in one's belly," meaning one can persuade oneself of anything.

J. Avni (Israel).   I found the presentation by Dr. Moses interesting, but I believe it could also demonstrate the dangers of a psychoanalyst going into politics. We have to ask ourselves whether a psychoanalyst can be objective enough if he has political views. Does he have the tools to judge things scientifically? Could he not be using the same mechanisms of projection, splitting, and projective identification, dividing people into the good guys and the bad guys? We have heard a discussion that involved one political point of view, but what about the views of those at the other extreme?

Unidentified speaker (Israel).   There are parts of the world where people of different religions, who even speak different languages, live side by side in relative harmony. The classic example is Switzerland, but in other places, such as Northern Ireland or India, they are killing one another. Is there some way we can use the principles that have been described to explain these differences?

Otto Kernberg.   I very much enjoyed the application of the concepts of projection and projective identification to the political process as we heard it today. In illustrating how these concepts are applied, Dr. Moses has helped us find some definitions with which we might all be able to live, which can help us bring together the different views of such concepts as identification, projection, and projective identification. I hadn't thought about this before, but I would like to suggest as a working hypothesis that we all tend to use the same terms in weak and strong senses. In a weak sense we use the term projection for the attribution of something internal to something outside. I don't think anyone would disagree with that. The weak use of the term is the most general, and the term is an umbrella one. It includes projection onto the leader of the horde, the large group, as Freud suggested, as well as referring to the transference in general terms. And then we use the term projection, and also projective identification, in a strong sense, with very specific, circumscribed meanings. Now of course projective identification can also be used in a weak sense, but I think it would be better to use projective identification only in the strong one as a very specific mechanism, as part of the umbrella term. The same may be true for introjection, which we use in a way that is so broad that it is almost the equivalent of internalization, particularly primitive internalization. But introjection has more specific meanings when used in a strong sense. This conference has not been about introjection, but I think the distinction between the weak and strong senses would probably also apply. Finally, the same is true for identification, which I think we have been using in a weak sense, in the sense that one becomes changed in some way on the model of something other than oneself. I suppose everyone would agree with that, but identification in a strong sense has more specific requirements. We speak of partial identification, selective identification, identification involving a higher level of introjection, and so on.

I should like to support the point made by Dr. Berman, who pointed out that the ideal leader has to absorb the need of the masses but then has to return it to them in a functional way. This is an important aspect of leadership. The leader has to be able to see what the needs of the group are but at the same time has to maintain awareness of external reality, so that emotional needs can be transformed into a realistic program. This is in contrast to either simply rejecting emotional needs or simply accepting them fully. It is a very interesting concept. The comment made by Dr. Stelzer about rigidity and extremism also applies, because sometimes we call those who are on the opposing pole of the spectrum extreme. That is a fair criticism, and it is true that only the leaders of the right were mentioned. I thought I could read Dr. Moses's political views in his statement. I am not saying that I disagree with them, but I think that we cannot have it both ways as psychoanalysts. Either we try to do a technical analysis which forces us to be politically neutral for the time being, or else we use psychoanalysis as a way of promoting our own views. This sort of thing is what liquidated the Marxist analysis of political ideology; that analysis is a class-determined rationalization of the political needs of a certain social class. This necessarily led to Marxism as a political ideology, as the ideology of the working class, and therefore led it into relativism. This was incompatible with Marxism considered as the scientific approach to reality. As psychoanalysts we should not fall into the same trap. Let me play devil's advocate for a moment, and let us say that I am the rightist side of Dr. Moses, and am applying his analysis to leftist leadership. One could say that there exists a leader who uses the split-off idealization and denial of aggression, and who says, "Look, we Jews should be morally superior. We can't treat the Arabs like they treat us. We have an historical, cultural, and religious mission and if we don't live up to that morality we don't deserve to exist." There are eminent Jews, coming from a strong Jewish background, who have dedicated their political life with enthusiasm and courage to attacking Israel at every point, and to ignoring anything wrong with the Arabs. If five thousand people are killed by the Syrians, then that is understandable because that is how the Arabs are, but the events of

Sabra and Shatilla are crimes against humanity. I am not defending any of these barbarous occurrences, but I want to draw attention to the fact that we can have the good leader, the morally ideal one, who projects aggression and unconsciously achieves a brutal attack on the survival of Israel. So I think we have to be very careful. I think that Dr. Moses probably agrees with me.

We need, from a psychoanalytic viewpoint, to differentiate crowds and masses from large groups. When Freud spoke about group psychology he was talking about mass psychology or crowd psychology. Much of the recent psychoanalytic literature is, by contrast, about large groups, which are groups of between forty and say a hundred and fifty people, in which there is still some communication possible. But Dr. Moses has talked more about masses, temporarily activated crowds and political communities, rather than large groups in the technical sense. This is perhaps a minor point, but because so much of psychoanalytic literature is emerging using the concept of the group differently, it is useful to make the differentiation. The leadership of masses or mobs or political communities has, I think, characteristics that are quite close to what Freud described in his book on group psychology, but what Freud neglected was a phenomenon that has been called the static crowd in contrast to the dynamic one. Dr. Moses talked about the dangers of the leader who doesn't absorb aggression, and we can see this particularly in the leader of the dynamic crowd, the crowd that is going to go out and do something, to smash, destroy, or fight. But in contrast there is a more static crowd that is happy and wants to be left alone, and that crowd usually selects as a leader a quiet, self-satisfied narcissist who feeds them, who looks very flexible and friendly on the surface, who serves as a superficial cliché with which everyone is happy because everyone understands it. This avoids the unconscious envy of the individual who thinks independently, and the unconscious envy of individuality and creativity, the unconscious envy of the leader as a powerful force.

Rafael Moses. Dr. Székely wondered why it is that only Jewish men were demonized while Jewish women were described as pleasant and agreeable. He pointed out that this is a state of affairs that has existed since the Middle Ages. I think this is understandable if we keep in mind that it was the Jewish men who were the main representatives of the group toward the outside. In the Nazi ideology, too, the focus was on Jewish men: the men were considered dangerous. However, the Nazi ideology also illustrates what is important about the women of the enemy, Jewish or otherwise. They are dangerous in that they may be attractive to men of the supposedly superior group. Such an attraction would then work against the desired separation of the two groups. I tend to think that then, as now, the women of the enemy are for this reason *not* described or regarded as pleasant, even when the main focus is not on them.

The idea that the qualities of a small group from the enemy population is extrapolated to the whole group is, I believe, a widespread phenomenon in prejudice and enmity of any kind. We find it both within a society and in the enmity between two peoples.

The comment that there are three types of leader rather than two—by analogy to the three types of analyst—is very interesting. Yet I think that while there are three groups, there are only two types. Certainly an analyst or a leader may leave what is projected into him untouched. He may do so either by rejecting it outright or by, as it were, swallowing it whole. In neither case does he mute the disturbing material. It is only when he can accept it within himself, and then mitigate or mute it, that the mother, the leader, or the analyst can use projective identification in order to bring about positive and therefore moderating change. This change will then be beneficial both for the projector and for his surroundings. I tend to think that this applies equally to the political left and to the right; and, of course, to the middle too.

The question of whether what is projected falls on fertile ground—i.e., increases feelings, attitudes, or wishes that are already present—is an interesting one. I think we should look at this more. Yet I can well imagine that even in a supervisory group of therapists, when a feeling is transmitted by talking about a patient who is not known to the group, the feelings about the patient may be experienced on the basis of existing feelings. Perhaps this is connected with the degree to which we are ready to expose ourselves to feelings and to become aware of them.

The point was made by several speakers that I seem to be in danger of misusing my psychoanalytic tools in order to bring out or strengthen a one-sided political view. I certainly agree that this is a danger that one should keep in mind. I also think it quite likely that my political views did show. And I agree that it would be better if they did not. But the real danger, to my mind, is that these tools are used so one-sidedly that they cannot equally be applied to the other side. I think one also has to bear in mind the fact that the government in power is the one that is usually looked at; and this is what I did. I certainly do think that this way of looking at a political situation can—and should—be equally applied to both sides. So Dr. Kernberg's example is certainly no less one-sided. It makes the leftist leader appear totally unaccepting of his own aggression.

But in fact leaders on both sides are not all that one-sided, as I think I was trying to point out. But it is certainly worth our while to develop a study of the Israeli left. I hope it will be done.

I think we have a similar situation as far as extremism and rigidity is concerned. Political extremism is ordinarily rather well-defined. I would not include in it a situation that requires self-defense, such as that which existed in Israel in 1948; nor does it seem right to me that we should discard the term extremism in favor of rigidity. After all, we are here considering political behavior as the independent variable, and personality aspects as the dependent ones. What must come to mind in this context is the much discussed fact that we would not want people to be so good at adapting to an intolerable situation that they would support its continuation. That, it seems to me, is the other side of the coin.

Joseph Sandler. I want to interrupt you at this point and ask Dr. Mibashan if she can put her point more precisely and explain Dr. Grinberg's concept of projective counteridentification. You could then integrate that into your response.

Naomi Mibashan. I am sorry I was not clear enough, but Grinberg's concept is really a very difficult one to explain and to understand. In your paper, Dr. Moses, you speak of the predisposition of the receiver of a projective identification. I wanted to call attention to the fact that it is not necessary that the receiver have a predisposition to act in the way the sender wants him to, to have the same tendencies as the split-off and projected aspects the other person is trying to put into him. I gave the example of a group supervision in which a group of eight therapists might be listening to an account that had produced an unconscious reaction, a projective counteridentification in the therapist; they then feel the same reaction, the same projective counteridentification, but it must be clear that these eight people do not necessarily all have the same predisposition. They may have, but it is not a necessary condition. A therapist may feel all kinds of things in reaction to a patient's projective identification. He may feel confused, he may feel angry. He may feel impotent or guilty.

Rafael Moses. Thank you, it is very clear.

I was delighted by the comment about Switzerland. If we knew how to turn Israel into Switzerland we would all be very happy, but I don't think we know enough to do that.

Dr. Kernberg's comments on the weak and strong senses in regard to the concepts of projection, projective identification, introjection, and identification are most interesting, and certainly worth thinking about much more. However, I want to respond particularly to Dr. Kernberg's comments about crowds and mobs. When I was talking about large groups I was not thinking of a mob in the sense of a large crowd listening to a speaker, or being led by someone in conditions under which it is easy for the crowd to be induced to action that can be quite dangerous. I would differentiate quite clearly such a crowd or mob, a large group of people coexisting at a given point in time and space, with a leader who is present, from a large group such as a stratum within our society or a part of a nation or people, who represent a group but do not congregate physically at the same point in space and time.

Lars Sjögren (Sweden).   I have been somewhat confused by the use of the concept of projective identification during the conference, as it has been loosened from its Kleinian context. This has resulted in a difficulty because we have a sort of confusion of tongues, with many people trying to take this Kleinian concept and push it into another context. This is, of course, one of the great problems we have in psychoanalysis today—the problem of creating some kind of common language without destroying the different contributions coming from the various schools. This is an enormous task for us.

I want to say something about the concept of projective identification, which really belongs in the paranoid-schizoid position. It is from that position that the mechanism is used, and it is the paranoid-schizoid position that has to be lived through in order for the individual to find his identity. Projective identification necessarily goes with this process, and if one tries to enter the depressive position prematurely, one will enter a confusional state, or one in which creativity is killed in some way. I think that there is a parallel here in relation to groups and nations, as they also have to go through this process. One can see that a premature attempt to enter the depressive position can then bring about confusion or death—I am thinking of death in the sense of spiritual death. Some Jewish friends of mine have recently returned to their Jewish identity in a way that would have been unthinkable ten or fifteen years ago. At that time they were trying to be world citizens, and we can now see that that was premature. In a sense they tried to leave the paranoid-schizoid position too early. I want to say that I am not talking about the paranoid-schizoid position in a pathological sense, but rather as part of the process of finding an identity. The problem that often arises is that the paranoid feelings have to be controlled so that one does not become destructive. It is the problem of how to find an identity and not be destructive, even if this evokes paranoid feelings about others. We can see how this operates within religions. For example, we can see how different Christian churches carry different gifts to humanity and how different Jewish traditions within the Jewish culture bear different contributions. We cannot prematurely push all of this together as certain ecumenical enthusiasts want us to do. We have to accept that the splits between the groups are not necessarily something terrible. They also represent a way of keeping up special traditions. So we face the problem within religions, within politics, within nations, and between nations, of keeping our identities and letting the others keep their identities, while still coming to terms with one another. Of course we can only hope that this sort of thing might be possible before we are all blown up in some sort of final catastrophe. I was reminded, when someone mentioned Switzerland, that Harry Lime, the Third Man, says in the film of that name that Switzerland had peace for four hundred years, and what did they produce? Cuckoo clocks! So that is the problem for us—how to tolerate conflict sufficiently and not go into some sort of confusional state or the death of creativity that Harry Lime talks about.

Rafael Moses. Thank you Dr. Sjögren. Let me just say that I think some of us in Israel would like to be known only for cuckoo clocks. But, more seriously, this conference seems to me to be about understanding all these concepts, particularly the concept of projective identification. It is a Kleinian idea, but I don't think we have to accept the whole Kleinian theory in order to understand it and perhaps make use of it. Speaking as someone who, as I said in my paper, was not brought up on projective identification in my psychoanalytic training, I still think it is a useful concept in many ways. But I cannot accept the theoretical view Dr. Sjögren just put forward. I am not a party to Melanie Klein's way of understanding early childhood and the mechanisms that are thought to be used then. Yet the concept of projective identification has very useful applications. Perhaps we can at some time look more at the things that go on between the separate groups of people—those who have accepted projective identification and those who have not, and possibly come to terms a bit more with each other.

Joseph Sandler. For those who are worried that one cannot ingest some form of projective identification, no matter how it is cooked and served up, so to speak, without ingesting the whole of Kleinian theory, let me say that there are antecedents to this concept. The concept was a felicitous formulation by Melanie Klein in 1946, and she certainly added something of her own, but she added something to an already existing concept. In 1936 Anna Freud had introduced a number of defense mechanisms which involved the idea of transpositions of self and object. She spoke about identification with the aggressor, about altruistic surrender, and so on. Melanie Klein's concept crystallized something which was very important and very much in the air, even among those who did not agree with Kleinian theory. But her formulation obviously had a great impact. What the discussion has drawn attention to is how much of what we do in relation to others is connected with the way we dispose of aspects of ourselves and of our objects, and how there are important processes of moving the representations of these around in different situations. This is not only a developmental process but something we do in the present as well, and although we might disagree with some of the specific formulations which have been put forward, in general this way of thinking about the rearrangement of aspects of representations of self and object is a relatively new one in psychoanalysis, and very important from the point of view of our theory of object relationships. It will certainly influence the development of analysis in the future, and has application outside the analytic sphere, as Rafael Moses has shown us today.

Chapter 11

Dybbuk Possession and Mechanisms of Internalization and Externalization: A Case Study

YORAM BILU *

As indicated by other contributors to this volume, psychoanalysts differ markedly in the importance they ascribe to projective identification as a special psychic mechanism. While some of them have welcomed the introduction of this concept by Melanie Klein (1946) as a major contribution to post-Freudian psychoanalysis, others tend to devalue its clinical significance or to consider it altogether redundant to its antecedents, projection and identification. The fact that projective identification is a controversial concept in clinical practice, its own natural habitat so to speak, may lead to the conclusion that efforts to apply it to other nonclinical spheres should be discouraged altogether. Yet in some realms such remote applications may lend us valuable insights as to processes underlying phenomena far removed from the analytic couch. An example in case is Rafael Moses's discussion of the political process in this volume.

The focus of the work presented here is the interface between psychology and anthropology. It discusses the peculiar career of a Jewish woman in a nineteenth-century Eastern European Hasidic community, a career ended by an episode of dybbuk possession. Although the details of this episode were not specified in the account that is drawn on, the case was selected for presentation because, unlike most other reports of this Jewish variant of spirit possession, it contains significant information concerning the social matrix in which it evolved, as well as the biographies of its main protagonists. On the basis of this information an attempt will be made to render the possession episode intelligible in terms of the psychodynamic and sociocultural factors underlying it. Although various

163

concepts of internalization and externalization are employed in this work (without being accorded a ubiquitous status), it is particularly projective identification which seems intriguingly related to spirit possession. This relationship will be specified after a brief review of the historical, theosophical, and sociocultural aspects of the dybbuk. Later, in the concluding section, the case under study will be discussed in terms of internalization and externalization.

DYBBUK POSSESSION AND EXORCISM

While case studies of spirit possession in various cultures are well represented in the anthropological literature (Obeyesekere, 1970; Crapanzano and Garrison, 1977; Goodman, 1981), the dybbuk has been the exclusive domain of creative writers such as Ansky (1926) and Singer (1959). The reason for this lack of scientific investigation is twofold: first, although dybbukim (the plural form) thrived in many Jewish communities as early as the sixteenth century (Scholem, 1971), the general disintegration of the Jewish traditional centers in Europe and the Middle East in our time has eliminated them altogether. As a result, no contemporary cases of dybbuk possession have been available since the 1930s. Second, the bulk of dybbuk accounts are to be found in mystically oriented exegeses of the Scriptures, in books of Hasidic tales and in special booklets and brochures, written either in Rabbinical Hebrew or in Yiddish. Evidently these sources remain inaccessible to many scholars. Recently this predicament was partially rectified by a scholar in Judaic studies who meticulously collected and annotated many reports of dybbuk possession (Nigal, 1983). In the absence of in vivo cases, however, the methodological problem of relying on secondary sources, written from a definite moral and religious perspective, remains quite compelling. The case analysis that ensues is not exempt from this disadvantage, as it concerns a dybbuk episode that occurred long before the author of the account on which it is based was born. Yet this account is replete with details that enable a unique glimpse into the motivational level of the actors.

Dybbuk possession, by definition, involved spirits of the dead as possessing agents. Since these spirits were deemed malevolent and dangerous, the phenomenon was conceived of as a disease, for which exorcism, performed by a rabbi-healer, was considered the only remedy. Unlike many other cultures (Lewis, 1971; Bourguignon, 1973; Crapanzano and Garrison, 1977), Judaism did not possess the positive category of ceremonial possession, in which the dissociative state is not stigmatized but socially approved, and the adept seeks to establish a symbiotic relationship with the possessing agent (Bilu, 1980, p. 36). The ideational matrix in which the dybbuk phenomenon germinated was the mystical doctrine of transmigration of souls (*gilgul*), formulated as early as the twelfth century (Scholem, 1971), but developed into a universal law during the sixteenth century. Specifically, it was the concept of impregnation (*ibbur*), derived from that doctrine, that laid the theosophical basis for possession by elaborating the possibility of a spirit's penetrating a living person *after* he was born (whereas transmigration supposedly occurs at conception or birth). The designation dybbuk, derived from the Hebrew verb *davok*, to stick, was applied to spirits who penetrated humans in order to find refuge from celestial persecutions. Since these were the spirits of notorious sinners, they were doomed to remain in limbo, without even being allowed entrance to hell (where spirits could be purged and proceed toward heaven). In this liminal state they were exposed to relentless torments inflicted upon them by angelic and demonic beings. Inhabiting humans provided these persecuted spirits temporary shelter, which they were unwilling to leave unless forced to through harsh exorcistic measures.

Since the theosophical doctrines underlying the dybbuk concept were formulated within the framework of Jewish mysticism, it is no wonder that this Jewish variant of possession appeared mainly in mystically oriented circles, Sephardic as well as Ashkenazi. Most of the early cases, in the sixteenth and seventeenth centuries, were documented in Italian and Middle Eastern Sephardic communities, but during the eighteenth and nineteenth centuries East European Hasidic communities, mainly in Russia and Poland, supplied most of the reports.

As in other cultural variants of possession (Oesterreich, 1930; Lewis, 1971; Walker, 1972; Bourguignon, 1976), women were clearly overrepresented among the dybbuk victims, whereas most of the possessing spirits were male. Thus the most prevalent pattern of gender combination among the dybbukim was a male spirit penetrating a female human. This pattern may be accounted for by the "deprivation hypothesis" (Lewis, 1966, 1971; Greenbaum, 1973), as a form of female protest: i.e., in a male-dominated society, the idiom of spirit possession enables a troubled woman to borrow a potent masculine identity through which behaviors normally proscribed to her may be acted out in a socially acceptable way. An alternative explanation may consider spirit possession a very convenient metaphor for articulating experiences related to female sexuality (Bourguignon, 1981): the fact that the victim is penetrated by the possessing agent coincides with the female's traditionally receptive role during coitus, while the very state of possession, in which an external entity resides in the victim's body, bears a clear resemblance to pregnancy. In the documented cases of dybbukim sexual overtones are quite salient. They are manifested, among other things, in the conceptual formulations of possession (e.g., the doctrine of impregnation), in the selection of the vagina as a preferred site of penetration, in the verbalized motivations of the spirits to take possession of their victims, and in their transgressions during their lifetime, confessed during the exorcistic ritual. (For a fuller discussion of the sexual aspects of dybbuk possession, see Bilu, 1985.) In addition to sexuality, however, the dybbuk idiom served as an outlet for other urges and desires, some of which are clearly related to the "deprivation hypothesis." In fact, as these explanations are more complementary than exclusive, both might apply to many of the case reports, including the one to be analyzed later.

Dybbuk possession is depicted through the case reports as a crystallized syndrome, the behavior patterns of which remain relatively stable across time and space. Although the literary promulgation of the cases might have contributed to this uniformity, it should be remembered that the symptoms were not idiosyncratically construed, but rather derived their form and meaning from a public set of symbols shared by most members of the community. During the possession episode, which was characterized by altered consciousness and later masked by amnesia, the inhabiting spirit's presence was clearly felt through odd bodily postures, violent convulsions, strange vocalizations, obscene verbalizations, and self- and other-directed aggressive behaviors. Xenoglossia, divination, and mastery of specialized skills were also common spirit-specific behaviors.

As in other cultural variants of possession-as-disease (Oesterreich, 1930, p. 103), the exorcism of the dybbuk was construed as a patterned sequence of steps, the strict following of which perforce culminated in its expulsion. Through these steps the spirit's identity and posthumous vicissitudes were disclosed, the conditions for its departure negotiated, and the body site through which it would eventually leave (usually one of the big toes) agreed upon (Patai, 1978; Bilu, 1980). The exorcist, usually a mystically oriented rabbi, executed his interventions in a fixed, gradual order, escalating from milder measures of verbal coaxing of the spirit to adjurations and decrees of excommunication. Coercive methods of fumigating the dybbuk or beating it were resorted to after verbal alternatives had been exhausted and found ineffective. Often the exorcism was performed in the synagogue with the active participation of a *minyan* (a religious quorum of ten male adults), or even the entire audience. In this setting, Jewish sacred paraphernalia (Torah scrolls, ritual horns, candles) were employed during the critical stages of the exorcism in order to facilitate the expulsion of the spirit.

Not surprisingly, the exorcistic ritual has been the rhetorical climax in most of the case accounts. The rabbi-spirit encounter was usually depicted as a long and bitter struggle, emotionally charged and exhausting. The healer had to mobilize all his stamina and resourcefulness to overcome his insidious adversary, for whom, it should be recalled, the victim's body constituted a longed-for refuge from incessant and merciless persecution. Notwithstanding this dramatization, the exorcistic ritual appears as a most successful psychotherapy. Judging from the reported cases, most of the possessed were completely and irreversibly cured.

Beyond this individual aspect of control, the elaborate cultural processing and the rich moralistic implications of the dybbuk has made it a very powerful vehicle for enhancing obedience in the community at large. Particularly the spirits' terrible sufferings in the hereafter, minutely described by them during exorcism, provided evidential confirmation for the idea that in the coming world, regulated by principles of reward and punishment, the righteous are prosperous and the wicked are doomed. In many cases the immediate effects of these recountings were so striking as to produce deep sentiments of compunction and repentance in the entire audience. In this way symptoms representing deviant motivations, which, if directly expressed, would have been quite disruptive to the fabric of Jewish life, were transformed into a conformity-enhancing device.

<h2 style="text-align:center">SPIRIT POSSESSION AND CONCEPTS OF
INTERNALIZATION AND EXTERNALIZATION</h2>

The dybbuk and other forms of spirit possession may be psychodynamically construed as a peculiar interplay of internalization and externalization. This interplay, however, does not fit in with standard definitions of projective identification. In certain aspects, if we follow Kernberg's criteria for differentiating projection from projective identification (see Chapter 7), the dybbuk clearly appears to be a manifestation of the former. Elsewhere I have addressed myself in detail to the unacceptable intrapsychic materials, mainly of a sexual but also of an aggressive nature, that are projected onto the object—the spirit—in the case of the dybbuk (Bilu, 1985). In line with Kernberg's definition of projection there seems to be lack of empathy with the projected contents, as well as estrangement from the object. This estrangement, however, is not accompanied by physical distancing. Rather, conversely, the dybbuk dynamics involve a bidirectional flow: what is projected is also taken in. The latter, inward-oriented motion constitutes a form of internalization, albeit a most concrete and "primitive" one.

A peculiar aspect of the dybbuk as an integrated process of externalization and internalization is that, epistemologically, these two concepts are not located on the same level. Whereas projection is a purely inferred process, its inward-directed counterpart takes a very concrete form of which all the participants are amply aware. This discrepancy stems from the special ontological status ascribed to spirits in many cosmologies of non-western societies, which makes them capable of invading humans in a most literal sense. Whereas for a native participant, estranged from psychoanalytic reasoning, the idea of the spirit as a "container" for the victim-to-be's projected experiences would seem utterly untenable, he would readily espouse the contrasting, "empirically based" notion of the victim being the container of the invading spirit. This position, however, is not diametrically opposed to that of a psychodynamically oriented social scientist who, while denying the credulous notion of possession-as-literal-introjection, would otherwise try to reformulate it on a metaphorical level: it is not the object but rather its representation that is "being taken in." Since this object representation is actually a self-representation, we notice here a peculiar process of projection turned inward.

The fact that the representations projected onto the object are personified though an internally located (though ego-alien) entity has far-reaching consequences concerning attempts to control the object— an important aspect of the differential definition of projective identification. Whereas from the native's point of view the possessed appears as a passive victim who cannot exert control over the spirit even to a minimal degree, a psychodynamic reading would not fail to recognize the ample opportunity given to the possessed to act out projected aspects of his self under the idiomatic cover of the spirit. Since possession is a cultural device through which an intrapsychic conflict is assigned an "interpersonal" dimension, evoking the projected behavior in the spirit-as-object is far more effective than in manifestations of projective identification reported in clinical practice.

THE CASE OF EIDEL: DESCRIPTION AND EXEGESIS

The dybbuk account under discussion is taken from the memoirs of an Israeli scholar of Judaic studies, dedicated to his childhood in the

Galician town of Brody (Sadan, 1938). Prior to World War I, Brody was an important Jewish center, located on the border between the Austro-Hungarian Empire and Czarist Russia. As a child, Sadan had heard many stories concerning the Jewish community of his hometown during earlier generations, which he later set down in his book. One of these stories was the account of a peculiar case of a dybbuk that had taken possession of a woman named Eidel in the second half of the nineteenth century. The account was related to him by his grandmother, who claimed to have been an eyewitness. A significant aspect of the case was the fact that it involved a highly venerated Hasidic family, the history of which is well documented. Therefore some of the details in the account (though not the dybbuk episode itself) could be corroborated through other sources.

From a psychodynamic perspective, the roots of the drama that culminated in Eidel's possession may be traced back to the formative years of her father, Rabbi Shalom Rokach, the founder of the well-known Hasidic sect of Belze. Rabbi Shalom (1783–1855) was born in Brody into a distinguished family, the genealogy of which included great sages and rabbinical scholars. When he was a small child, his father died and he was sent to another town to live with a maternal uncle. Hence, within a short while, young Shalom underwent two traumatic separations: having lost his father, he was then removed from his mother, to whom he was strongly attached. The fact that his mother, who stayed in Brody, soon remarried might have exacerbated his feelings of privation and loss. Under his uncle's patronage, however, these feelings were greatly mitigated. The uncle helped his young nephew to complete his rabbinical education under the greatest Hasidic masters of that time, and gave him his daughter Malka as a wife. From the outset, this marriage proved extraordinarily harmonious. In the text, the motivational basis for Rabbi Shalom's boundless love for his wife was explicitly linked to his sentiments toward his mother: "Evidently, his longings for his mother, which inflamed his soul, were displaced onto the luminous figure of his noble cousin." If, indeed, the close union of marriage constituted for Rabbi Shalom a compensation for the separation from his mother, then selecting the *maternal* cousin as a substitute love object seems suggestive. While such a "psychological" idea was not entertained by the official chronicles of the Belze sect, they also took great pains to stress the mutual affection and devotion that prevailed in the relationship of the couple. This profound attachment persisted in later years in Belze, where Rabbi Shalom's growing reputation as a great Hasidic master and spiritual authority granted him thousands of devoted followers from all over Galicia. His adherents, who referred to him as *admor* (a Hebrew acronym for "our master, teacher, and rabbi"), considered him a *tsaddik* (a pious, holy man) and flocked to his court asking for advice, blessing, and remedy. The intimate, harmonious relations between Rabbi Shalom and his wife were noted by many visiting rabbis, one of whom found the couple, then in old age, "like Adam and Eve before the sin" (Klepholtz, 1972, p. 86).

This affectionate bond was tragically broken with the sudden death of the Rabbi's wife, which left him heartbroken and dejected. Once again he was deprived of a love object to whom he was fervently attached. For many years he could not be consoled, refusing to accept God's verdict and entreating him to bring his beloved spouse back to life. His only ray of comfort in this anguish was his daughter Eidel, the third significant female figure in his life.

Of Rabbi Shalom's five sons and two daughters, Eidel, the younger girl, was clearly his favorite. It might be speculated that she won most of her father's affection, despite the strong cultural preference for male descendants, because for him she was an extension of her mother and grandmother, whom she replaced as an object of libidinal investment. However, Rabbi Shalom could not ignore the substantial disadvantages of being born female in a society where "women are accorded less importance than men" (Mintz, 1968, p. 83). Eidel's femininity, a guaranteed prescription for inferior status and exclusion from spiritual and intellectual life (Lacks, 1980, p. 163), was for Rabbi Shalom a predicament to which he could not reconcile himself. The resultant tone of unrelieved wistfulness which colored the Rabbi's admiring attitude toward Eidel found expression in the text as follows: "He [Rabbi Shalom] said: the preserved light that should have illuminated the whole world is contained in my daughter Eidel. If she were male, she could have hastened the coming of salvation. No one could be as pious. It was due to Satan's mischievous interference that she was not born male." That Rabbi Shalom repeatedly tried to rectify this interference shows the same wishful yearning to change what is irrevocable as had occurred in his reaction to his wife's death.

As Zborowski and Herzog (1962) ornately describe, raising a daughter as a son was a rare phenomenon, limited to a specific family constellation: "If there is no son to be a *kheider* [religious school] boy, to be examined on a Sabbath afternoon, to shed luster and inflame pride by his recitations, a father may so yearn for an intellectual heir that he will try to build up his daughter into one" (p. 128). Since Rabbi Shalom had five potential intellectual heirs, Eidel's higher position may be viewed on the manifest level as a sheer expression of her father's love and care, in the context of the male-oriented Jewish communities of former centuries. Yet in the intimate, tacit context of a "family romance" it might well reflect a defensive device against libidinal wishes and fantasies with regard to his daughter. (This is a paraphrase of Horney's discussion of the masculinity complex in women [1926]. In accord with the oedipal paradigm, Horney attributed these wishes to the daughter.)

Rabbi Shalom's pathetic attempts to masculinize Eidel were lucidly manifested in various symbolic gestures he made to adorn her with male religious artifacts. When she was young he would decorate her head with his phylacteries and skull cap, male ritual objects which convey a strong masculine phallic quality (Eder, 1933; Bilu, 1979, p. 450). Among the gifts he sent her after she had married and settled in Brody (his own native town) was a magnificent silk cover for a Torah scroll. When Eidel sent it back, assuming that he had mistaken it for a silk scarf, Rabbi Shalom made it clear that his present was properly conceived. "Is my Eidel not a Torah Scroll?" he asked, again using a common masculine metaphor usually employed to honor a male child. In his last moments, Rabbi Shalom pronounced his attitude toward Eidel directly and forcefully. When his daughters were removed from his death bed lest their excessive weeping and groaning spoil the moment of dying, the moribund rabbi persisted, "Eidel should stay, since for me she is not a daughter but rather a son."

After Rabbi Shalom's death, his youngest son, Rabbi Yeoshuah, inherited his throne and led the Belze sect for almost forty years, until the last decade of the nineteenth century. Eidel, for her part, managed to attract some of her father's followers, who admired her wisdom and erudition. They would come to her court in Brody asking for advice and blessings, and enjoyed her brilliant commentaries on the Torah. Evidently she functioned as an *admor* for these Hasidim, among whom she was known as Eidel the Rabbi.[1] In a society in which a woman rabbi was a role combination of the utmost incompatibility, this epithet should have been quite extraordinary. Whether one accepts that "there is no better sex in the Jewish religion," as orthodox apologetics contends (Appleman, 1979, p. 6), or that Jewish women were denied "the very essence or breath of human being," as modern feminists claim (Lacks, 1980, p. 165), it is evident that "women were excluded from scholarship study of the Torah and the obligatory, positive commandments that assured the Jewish spiritual and communal life" (Lacks, 1980, p. 125). As a result, the role of rabbi

[1]Sadan's grandparents were Eidel's adherents, and it is their version of her story which is presented here. In the official chronicles of the Belze sect, it was noted that she behaved like a rabbi, but the social drama which evolved from this behavior was entirely omitted.

seemed inaccessible to women. Still, the emergence of Eidel as an *admor* was not unprecedented. Jewish sources present an impressive if exiguous gallery of women who, since the Talmudic era, have pursued the role of religious scholar or religious functionary, both in Ashkenazi and Sephardic communities. Although never officially ordained as rabbis,[2] these women assumed important congregational positions, serving as leaders in synagogues, as teachers in religious academies, as scribes and commentators on the Torah, as ritual slaughterers, and also as *admors* in Hasidic communities, sometimes with their own established courts (Horodetsky, 1944; Alphasi, 1974).

The fact that Eidel lived in a Hasidic community is significant, since Hasidism seems to have been more conducive than other Jewish frameworks to the phenomenon of women rabbis. Hasidic sources refer to about fifteen women who behaved as *admors* (Alphasi, 1974). At least in its formative years in the eighteenth and nineteenth centuries, Hasidism was a mystically based movement with a clear social credo. It attracted the Jewish masses in Eastern Europe by offering them paths to God that did not rest on Talmudic scholarship and scholastic erudition. In so doing, it leveled a criticism against the rabbinical oligarchy, which considered these virtues tantamount to true religiosity. As a "religious movement of the oppressed," it seemed natural that women would be given a better status. Indeed, some reviews of Hasidism (especially that of Horodetsky, 1944) emphasized the egalitarian tendencies in the movement, noting the devaluation of formal study, the emergence of the *tsaddik* as a community leader accessible to both sexes, and the proliferation of popular Hasidic literature written in the vernacular (Yiddish) as the main developments that elevated women's status. In fact, these trends were either greatly idealized or else very short-lived, since, according to ethnographic evidence (Zborowski and Herzog, 1962; Mintz, 1968), the gap between the sexes in Hasidic sects has generally been preserved, and the exclusion of women from religious and spiritual life has not been significantly more lenient than in non-Hasidic circles. Therefore, even in Hasidic communities, where the significant nurturing dimension was added to the role of the *tsaddik*, and hence seems particularly fit for women, the phenomenon under discussion was deemed negligible and peripheral. This fact was manifested primarily in that women rabbis in Hasidism, as elsewhere,

---

[2] The first ordination of a woman to the rabbinate took place in the U.S. in 1972. Since then, more than forty women of the Reform and Reconstructionist movements have been ordained. Orthodox Jews unequivocally reject the idea of a woman rabbi.

constituted a very select, homogeneous group clearly discernible by its high socioeconomic status. Like Eidel, most of them were the daughters of renowned rabbis and sages who were raised in an atmosphere of learning and piety, enjoying their fathers' high prestige and relatively liberated from mundane concerns. As a result they developed comparatively high expectations as to their future vocation and were given more elbowroom to pursue it. As mentioned before, some of these women, who were born into families with no male descendants at all, were raised as son-substitutes and intellectual heirs (most renowned in this subgroup were the daughters of Rashi, the great medieval commentator). Particularly in Hasidic cases there were allusions to the important role played by the distinguished fathers in legitimizing and preparing the psychological matrix for their daughters' aspirations. Already, the Besht (an acronym for Rabbi Israel Ba'al Shem-Tov), founder of the Hasidic movement (1700–1760), was said to have considered his daughter one of his students, while other *admors* identified in their daughters "sparks of holiness" and piety characteristic of a *tsaddik* (Ashkenazi, 1953).

The detailed account of the case of Eidel enables us to go beyond these general sociological and psychological variables to unfold the psychodynamics presumably underlying her emergence as a rabbi. In this case, the Rabbi's deep attachment to this daughter was accounted for in the light of his earlier relationships with his mother and wife, and his attempts to masculinize her were explicated as nurtured by a conscious yearning to furnish his beloved daughter a better lot in a male-dominated society, together with an unconscious warding-off of libidinal wishes and fantasies associated with her. It might be suggested that her special relationship with her father informed her that being loved is associated with being male. This association seems conducive to the development of a particularly intensified masculine complex, the alleviation of which may have required an alteration of her feminine self-image (see Horney, 1926; Edgcumbe, 1976). To what extent this dynamic was facilitated by Eidel's rejection of her mother as an object for identification is hard to say, since their relationship is not mentioned in the texts. Of course, the generally inferior status allotted to women in the culture, enhanced in this case by the father's prominent stance, might have contributed to this end. In addition, it seems plausible to assume that the younger Eidel was at the time of her mother's death, the stronger the impact of this event on deterring her from taking her mother as a role model.

In internalizing a male representation, Eidel probably followed the model set before her by her admired father. Whether or not she identified with him in the context of a negative oedipal phase, as a regressive yielding of the father as a love object, the idea that she created an introject of him is entertained in the light of subsequent episodes in her life. The first of these events was, of course, Eidel's attempt to follow in her father's footsteps by becoming an *admor*. There is some scant evidence in the Belze chronicles that in enacting this role she explicitly used Rabbi Shalom as a model, reiterating verbatim, for example, his healing formulae when ailing adherents came to her door. Moreover, Eidel did not rest content in her self-established court in Brody. Fortified by her deep conviction that she was her father's true heir and successor, she declared open war on her brother, the second *admor* of the Belze sect, accusing him of social injustice and corruption.

Sociologically, Eidel's reproaches should be understood in the context of the process of expansion and institutionalization that the Belze sect, as well as other Hasidic courts, underwent during the nineteenth century. Within an amazingly short time, Hasidism was transformed from an innovative social movement, persecuted for its mystical ideas, into the dominant force in Eastern European Jewry, an inseparable part of the orthodox establishment. In various settings, including Belze, this transformation was manifested in the contrast between the plain living and modesty of the founder of a Hasidic dynasty, and the affluence and haughtiness of the second generation, brought about by the mounting popularity of the *tsaddikim* and their exaltation to the level of sainted figures. Eidel's social pathos, however, might well have reflected a rekindling of infantile conflicts related to sibling rivalry. As Rabbi Shalom's favorite child, she believed herself to be the true carrier of his legacy and felt usurped by her brother. His affluent court all the more strengthened her conviction that he was altogether dissociated from their father's way of life and, hence, unentitled to his throne. Eidel's tragedy was that her personal conviction was not shared by the Hasidic communities in and around Belze. Her followers were few compared with the masses of her brother's adherents, mainly from the small shtetls and villages of Galicia. After all, she was only a woman, a fact that could be denied in fantasy life but not in the real world (see Lubin, 1958, for a discussion of similar dynamics in a case of a "feminine Moses"). That she nevertheless initiated a battle against her brother might be taken as an indication of how thoroughly she introjected her father and how strongly she was engulfed by his expectations.

The clash between the siblings escalated as Eidel's accusations became more bitter and poignant and their rendering obsessive. Eventually, sensing her impending defeat, she gradually sank into what the text calls "the dimness of melancholy." To her brother's followers her behavior appeared so bizarre and aberrant as to invoke the idea that she had fallen prey to a dybbuk.

We do not have enough information to determine whether Eidel did manifest symptoms typical of dybbuk possession at that phase, or whether she was arbitrarily so labeled in order to render her behavior explicable and to moderate its revolutionary impact. From a feminist perspective, it seems plausible that the Hasidic leadership responded to the challenge that Eidel's "female protest" posed by falsely charging her with evil-spirit possession, a fabrication tantamount to (though less disastrous in consequences) accusing women of witchcraft in post-Medieval Europe (Ben Yehuda, 1980). Yet even if the characterization of Eidel as one possessed was initially forced upon her, her later enactment of the dybbuk role was clearly personally motivated and caused much embarrassment to her brother and his supporters. Accepting the validity of dybbuk possession as a culture-specific Jewish syndrome (Bilu, 1985), I believe that Eidel could have found it a particularly convenient idiom for articulating her experiences on both the psychodynamic and the ideological levels. Supporting evidence for this argument may be drawn from the case of Eidel's contemporary, The Maiden of Ludmir (1815–1892), certainly the most famous woman rabbi of all times (Biber, 1946; Tversky, 1950).

In view of the typical Jewish female scholar, the Maiden was a deviant case in two respects. First, her family was from the rank and file, and not from the rabbinical oligarchy. As a result, she pursued her vocation without a parental model, although her father, a well-to-do merchant, furnished her with all the means for study. Second, the Maiden of Ludmir went further than any other woman rabbi in traditional circles in her attempts to pass as a man, observing, for example, commandments exclusively prescribed for males. Hers was a real "female protest" and, for a while, a very successful one, as she managed to draw to her court many thousands of Hasidim and, like Eidel, threatened the hegemony of the Ukrainian *admors*. Yet even in this extreme case no attempt was made to defy notions concerning traditional views of males and females in a modern feminist style. The Maiden's protest was purely an individual affair. Accepting as given the frailty inherent in the female nature, she managed to circumvent it by claiming to have been granted a male soul. This spiritual transformation, precipitated by a dramatic episode of disease and altered consciousness, supplied her with an acceptable rationalization for her unnatural, manlike manners. (She shrewdly embedded into the trancelike "conversion" episode the most renowned Ukrainian *tsaddik* as the one who handed her the new soul.) Loyal to this self-conception, the Maiden, unlike other female rabbis (including Eidel[3]) refused to get married, in order not to profane her soul. In fact, her decline began soon after she had been convinced by that Ukrainian *tsaddik* to quit the single state and find a husband.

Against the background of this self-generated rationale, the fact that the Maiden of Ludmir was considered by some rabbis among her opponents to be a victim of dybbuk possession should come as no surprise; nor should it be conceived of as an altogether arbitrary fabrication. Actually, the two explanations are structurally identical in that both contend that a male soul or spirit was residing in a female body. As noted before, these two types of possession are contained within the mystical doctrine of impregnation (*ibbur*). Content-wise, there was, of course, a crucial difference between them: dybbuk possession, instigated by an evil spirit, was considered an extremely negative state, while the Maiden's claim that her new spirit pertained to a *tsaddik* placed a positive value on her transformation. The same controversy concerning the nature of the possessing agent evolved in the case of Eidel, to which we are now returning.

We have no information indicating that Eidel overtly entertained the idea that a male soul had been transplanted into her body; yet the fact that she was raised as a boy, pursued a male vocation, and presumably created an introject of her father seems to constitute a psychological climate conducive to the emergence of such an idea. Unlike the Maiden of Ludmir, however, Eidel did enact the role of the possessed, and in this enactment her hidden dialogue with her father was dramatically acted out.

In fact, the text depicts Eidel's possession only in the context of the exorcistic ritual, which took place before a large audience in a small town outside Brody. The exorcist was none other than her brother, Rabbi Yeoshuah, the second *admor* of Belze. This confrontation between the sibling adversaries made the emotionally charged episode of the exorcism all the more dramatic. But the mounting tension exploded ecstatically in the first stage of the meeting when, in response to the exorcist's routine

---

[3]In light of the present analysis, unfolding the nature of Eidel's marriage is of utmost importance, but the relevant information is extremely meager. It is noted, however, that Eidel's husband, an erudite rabbi, refused to behave as an *admor*, even though he was a descendant of a famous Hasidic master. This fact, contrasted with his wife's eagerness to be an *admor*, might be taken as an indication of a marital pattern in which the husband was passive and less domineering than his wife.

inquiry, Rabbi Shalom's flat voice burst out from Eidel's mouth. In front of the stunned audience the voice accused the exorcist of numerous transgressions, portraying the Belze court as an exemplar of vice and corruption. At first Rabbi Yeoshuah could not cope with these blatant reproaches, and retreated, embarrassed and humiliated. After a while, however, having redefined the possessing agent as an evil spirit who acted as an impostor, he recovered and resumed his attack on the dybbuk. For some time the exorcist's maledictions and adjurations intermingled with the spirit's charges and reproaches. Then the latter's low voice gradually faded away; the possessing agent, whether the father's spirit or an evil one, was exorcised, and Eidel, ostensibly cured by her brother, sank, according to the text, into the abyss of "complete darkness," never to regain her mental balance.

In light of the exegesis of Eidel's career, the dybbuk possession episode appears as an "appropriate" epilogue to her life drama. Having failed to realize her masculine strivings by dethroning her brother, she regressed from identifying with the father into a more primitive type of internalization, i.e., incorporation, a process "whereby the subject, more or less on the level of phantasy, has an object penetrate his body and keeps it 'inside' his body" (Laplanche and Pontalis, 1973, p. 211). By incorporating her father, Eidel resorted to the most extreme device supplied by her culture in order to assert, in a "visible," public manner, her linkage to Rabbi Shalom. For a short while, in fact, she and her father were one in a very concrete way. Her failure to substantiate her desperate claim, however, was followed by a total and irreversible collapse.

CONCLUSION

Eidel's dybbuk was depicted here as the end product of a strong masculine complex in a woman who was raised by her father as a male child and who subsequently pursued a male vocation, taking her father as a role model. In the possession episode, Eidel's strong identification with the father, heretofore inferred from her career as a rabbi, was manifested directly and lucidly. This affinity with the possessing agent makes Eidel's case very exceptional among the bulk of dybbuk accounts. Most of the other victims of possession, it should be recalled, have fallen prey to the spirits of complete strangers, usually notorious sinners, onto whom the most blatant antisocial wishes could be projected. Eidel's father, a pious and beloved Hasidic master, could hardly be used to that end.

Beyond this crucial difference in moral dimension, the case of Eidel uniquely involved an object that cannot be reduced to sheer fantasy (culturally endorsed and privately manipulated). Unlike other possessing spirits, Eidel's father existed on the level of ordinary reality, and his interactions with his daughter clearly had their effect on her later use of various modes of internalization. Can the father's behavioral attitude toward Eidel be translated into concepts of internalization and externalization? Without delving into the contents of his motivations (some of which were discussed earlier), the fact is that he grossly shaped the image of his daughter in line with his own fantasies. That he went as far as considering her a messianic harbinger may allude to some unattainable, wished-for grandiose self states as one unconscious source of his projection. (As a female, Eidel would have never been able to embody these strivings. That might have been one reason for the wish to masculinize her, but also, perhaps, for her selection as an object in the first place.)

If projective identification applies here at all, it seems to be operative at the interactive, interpersonal level (Zinner and Shapiro, 1972). Beyond *experiencing* the object as controlled by the projected parts of the ego, this case provides us an extreme example of the other being taken over and induced to respond in a manner dictated by the projection (Ogden, 1979). Eidel's display as a rabbi and as a dybbuk demonstrate the extent to which she was engulfed by her father's projected fantasies.

Chapter 12

Concluding Discussion

Joseph Sandler. We are certainly all very indebted to Dr. Bilu for his fascinating presentation. Of course, among psychoanalysts we also have many female rabbis, some of whom are possessed by the spirits of Sigmund Freud, Karl Abraham, Sandor Ferenczi, Melanie Klein, and others. We also have a form of exorcism, which is perhaps not quite as effective as the rabbinical one. And certainly, if we take the manifestations of xenoglossia, the use of strange and foreign languages, there is much evidence for demoniacal possession among some of our colleagues. However, on a more serious note, I think we have been shown very nicely how the projection of idealized, wished-for qualities can occur, and how these qualities can be forced into a receptacle that wants to have them. The question of the acceptance, by what we can call the projectee, of what the projector sends across is a crucial one in regard to the mechanisms we have been discussing.

Judith Issroff (Israel). We have all enjoyed the many attempts at clarifying the concepts of projective identification and projection. Unfortunately we have also heard how everyone uses a different kind of stance in conceptualizing, and this may lead to complete misunderstanding. I should like to look at the material we have just heard from another point of view. If we take the concept of learned helplessness, then the poor lady we have heard about, in her particular social context, could be said to have lapsed into a kind of protective silence. I think the concept of learned helplessness could be a very useful one.

We know that an interpretation can be made in such a way that the persecutory quality of the superego is increased, and this may lead to the production of the sort of phenomena we have seen from time to time in the clinical material that has been presented. Yet the same interpretation

179

might be made in another way, so that the persecutory or guilt-inducing quality of the superego is mitigated. The nature of the technique will determine the response in the patient. If we say that the analyst can experience what the patient is doing as a sort of attack, then perhaps the patient can also feel that he is being attacked, because of the way something is phrased.

Joseph Sandler.   I suspect that the lady described by Dr. Bilu was neither a poor lady, nor that she was experiencing learned helplessness. Perhaps we will get some comments on this.

Betty Joseph.   I would like to comment on one point. I think it is imperative in our discussion that we emphasize the importance of understanding the nature of the communication occurring between the patient and the analyst. Obviously we should try to become as sensitive as possible, not only to the effect that the patient has on the analyst, but also to the effect that the analyst and his or her interpretations have on the patient. I am very much in agreement with Dr. Issroff on this. But I think that what she refers to is exactly what we have all been talking about. In analysis a two-way process occurs, but it is of course extremely important that the analyst makes what we believe to be the correct interpretation. I mean "correct" in terms of what is going on in our relationship with the patient. We should not gloss over what we feel to be the truth in order to make it more palatable.

W. W. Meissner.   There is much to respond to, and I want to take one small element which may raise some methodological issues. As far as learned helplessness is concerned, we cannot equate learning something with internalization. This is my own point of view, and I am sure many would argue with it, but it seems to me there is a very big difference between what is learned and what is internalized. When we speak about internalization, using a psychoanalytic frame of references, we are not talking about something that is merely learned. A pertinent distinction in this area was made by David Rapaport when he contrasted the *inner* world with the *internal world*. The *inner* world was envisaged as being, in at least some of its aspects, as the representational world. It provided a kind of cognitive map by which the subject involved himself in the external world. By contrast, the *internal* world was seen by Rapaport as something different; it had to do with what became a part of the self-organization, a part of the psychic structure. It is in this realm that the notion of internalization has its meaning. I have used this as a basic supposition for my own thinking in this area. Now suppose an individual has had a series of experiences which provide a context of learning in which patterns of helpless behavior are acquired. That is something that can be observed and defined, but the psychoanalyst does not stop there. The psychoanalyst also asks whether there is something going on in the experience, perhaps step by step with the learning process, that speaks to an issue of internalization, that focuses on how the person's self-organization is constructed. This would dictate a need to take into account a realm of possible phenomena that had to do with how the person thinks, feels, and experiences in many dimensions. If we think of the case we have heard about from Dr. Bilu, we might well focus on the idea that she in a sense defined herself in a context of learned helplessness as a victim, and shaped her self-organization around that core, a process I would call introjective configuration. There are many different factors involved here, and as analysts we need to be careful that we don't settle for a piece of the pie when perhaps there is more to be eaten.

Otto Kernberg.   I would like to get back to the issue of our using a number of terms in somewhat different ways. I would guess that when the five of us at this table use some of these terms, we may give them slightly different meanings; at times the differences may be more than slight. Further, I think that when we use a number of terms, the way each of us organizes the whole constellation of terms varies. So if any one of us were asked whether we could say what is internalization, introjection, introjective identification, projection, projective identification, identity, partial identification, incorporation, and so on, and we were asked first whether all these concepts were somehow related, probably all five of us would say, "Yes, they are." If we were then asked to say how they are related, and what the differences are, each one of us would give different answers.

If I am correct, then a further point arises. As we talk about cases it becomes clear that the differences seem less terrible. The closer we get to clinical material, the more certain things tend to crystallize, and the differences between us become somewhat minor. This tempts us to turn to the clinical material and to say that good clinicians can understand each other, and that that is all that counts; theory is rather questionable; perhaps we can forget about theory and look into it later. Of course we *can* do that, and then everyone will be happy, but I want to resist the pressure to do this even at the risk of being called too abstract, too theoretical, and not sufficiently in touch with clinical practice. I want to take this stand because I think that although theorizing creates all sorts of nasty problems and confusions, it has the value that it can potentially generate new understanding and permit new ways of comprehending what we see clinically. It is an illusion to think that we only talk about what we see. All observations of clinical phenomena depend upon theories, and when we think that we are forgetting about theory, it only means that we have a theory of which we are not aware, which is sometimes nice and comfortable, but does not necessarily lead to scientific developments. I want to speak for the need to develop our theory, because this leads to new practical applications.

From this perspective it seems to me that there are two ways of proceeding. One is for each of us to spell out our underlying theory as fully as we can, and then to relate the way in which each of us defines all the concepts mentioned in relation to that theory. I think this would lead to clarification, although it would obviously be very time-consuming. It would lead to clarification because then everyone would know why we do have different ways of using these concepts, and why we organize them as we do. We would then find that we have differences in our theoretical approaches, and the next step might be that we would discuss these differences in our theories. That would be potentially creative if we were willing to listen to each other and to see where the points of contact are. Or we might go back to clinical phenomena, and then the differences in our understanding of them might be more meaningful. But whichever way we proceed, it is a long process. We don't have time for that, so it is the alternative road we must take. I want to say that we should accept certain definitions, as I have said, as weak ones, and others as strong ones, within the same conceptual line. Obviously this methodology comes from philosophy, where it has been used to deal with such concepts as the "categorical self," a strong concept which in philosophy corresponds roughly to our concept of identity. This is different from the weak concept of the self, in the sense of simple subjectivity or self-reflected subjectivity. It seems to me that there are three progressively stronger ways of talking about self—subjectivity, reflected subjectivity (more concise, stronger, and more delimited), and the categoric concept of the self. We might agree that in the broader sense projection includes both mechanism and outcome. It is both a mechanism of growth and adaptation and a mechanism of defense. Projection in the simplest sense consists of putting something outside which really belongs to the inside, of getting it out of oneself. Here it is a weak "umbrella" term, but it will become stronger when we circumscribe it to mean the projection of unacceptable impulses that are still recognized as such, are considered dangerous, and have to be controlled as they are projected onto another person; and the other person is then modified in the process. This is projective identification, roughly speaking. We can also talk about projection as attributing ideal parts of oneself to somebody else. Here we project but we don't reject what is projected. We identify with what is projected, as for example in projecting our ego ideal into the leader, projecting our superego and submitting to the leader, as Dr. Moses—following Freud—has described. And finally we can talk about projection as actualization in the transference. In other words, it is the projection of, for example, an object representation, and the activation of the relation with it. If I understood Dr. Meissner correctly, this is what he called displacement. Again, there may be a projection of an entire psychic structure, the id or the superego, and we are back to the first definition of projection of unacceptable impulses. Now in my view all these strong or categorical ways of using the concept of projection could be fitted under a weak concept with which we can communicate with one another while we try to specify the partial, stronger mechanisms such as projective identification. At this level, for example, I think that Betty Joseph and I would probably be largely in agreement in our definition of projective identification, although I would guess that she would be much less concerned about differentiating that from what I would call the weak umbrella concept, much more willing to put it together with other mechanisms without making strict differentiations. But I think that these problems are much less troublesome once we have agreed on the weak and strong terms.

The real differences between us are, however, at the level of theory. To say that projective identification is an exclusively Kleinian concept and cannot be used outside that context is not true. I think it can be used perfectly well in a different context, although the meaning will without doubt be affected. It seems to me that there are three basic questions in regard to which we have different viewpoints, and while I don't think they can be resolved here, I would like to spell them out. First, we can ask whether the birth of the human infant as a *psychological* being occurs at biological birth. Is there a separate psychic entity from the beginning or not? The answer for the Kleinians would basically be yes, and it evidently makes sense for them to talk about projection and introjection from the beginning. The same is probably true for Fairbairn, although he was somewhat ambiguous about that. On the other hand, for Winnicott and for Mahler, the answer is quite different. For Mahler, in particular, the birth occurs within a fused diadic state. This is as it is also seen by Harry Stuck Sullivan and Edith Jacobson. The second question is whether the human being, considered as a separate unit, is a one-person system. Or is it from the beginning a two-person system? And the third question is whether, if it is a fused merged system, it is all good, or a double-merged system, both for good and for bad. For Kohut, for example, the beginning of the system is an "all good" system, and there is a self, an all good, nonfragmented self. There is no such thing as a "bad" self. For most other authors the view is probably that at the beginning there is a simultaneously good and bad dyadic state. These are contrasting views that cannot be integrated here, but they make an enormous difference theoretically, because if one thinks that there is a separate self and object from the start, we can talk about projection and introjection from the beginning of life. If not, we have the task of deciding when we can talk about projection. What are the minimal developmental requirements? And if we consider that all internalizations are dyadic then we cannot say that one internalizes an object: one internalizes a relationship, and all the other definitions become more complicated. I could do the same thing with introjection that I have just done with projection. I could do the same for identification. I could give you a list of meanings, and could try to give a definition that has an umbrella meaning, but I am not interested in presenting a complete system here. Rather I want to find a way of communicating clinically without denying the differences in our theories, of keeping the richness of the discussion at the clinical level without using it to deny real theoretical differences that are important because they lead to scientific progress.

Rafael Moses.   I want to react to what Otto Kernberg has said. I am neither as catergorical as he is nor as hopeful when he implies that if we spell out our theoretical differences then we can convince one another, or come to see what would be a better way of conceptualizing. At conferences like this we listen to the others, but the question is always how much we take in. There may have been some slight changes in the views various people had about projective identification, but I am not at all sure that we have reached a position in which people will bring their disagreements out into the open. That would be the first step toward having a dialogue which would make for change on all sides.

Joseph Sandler.   I would add that it is probably not possible to get to a real dialogue in a meeting of this sort. However, I think it is possible that when we listen to someone else's notion of projective identification, we do identify, however fleetingly, with the other person. We might disidentify a moment later, but there is a sort of learning which can occur on the basis of that fleeting identification with the other person's point of view. If we can do anything at all to give the dialectic of development in this particular conceptual field a little shove, then this is a very good thing, and although we are very far from any closure (and I don't think we ought to have closure on this topic), then this is the most we can do. There can be no doubt that if the concept of projective identification, or even of projection or of identification, had been easily definable in theoretical terms we would not be having this discussion today. It is because we cannot get a good theoretical or even descriptive grip on the concept that we have the situation as it is. I am not sure that discussing the concepts at the theoretical level is as useful as Otto Kernberg regards it, but I would agree emphatically that by discussing things on the clinical level we get nearer to one another because the meaning of our concepts is so context-dependent. It is what surrounds the term in the description that gives it specific meaning, and we usually have no problem about understanding what a colleague means by introjection in a particular context, even though we might prefer to use the term identification in that context. If we climb to the theoretical heights we might discuss the matter till the cows come home, which is a very pleasant thing to do, of course, and I am sure that the subject will be discussed many times at that level; but I think it is the clinical material to which the concepts are anchored. Finally, I think Rafael Moses is right in that there may be people who are hesitant to voice their views. Perhaps we should make a greater effort to state our points of difference as clearly and as succinctly as possible.

M. Chayes (The Netherlands).   What I want to say may help to close the gaps between the theoretical and the clinical, because it concerns both. It may also serve to reduce somewhat the distinction between what happens before and after individuation. I refer here to the function of language as an instrument which can be empathically used to maintain or preserve cohesiveness and wholeness in the personality. This was illustrated very nicely in Betty Joseph's paper when she picked up, as the main communication of her patient N, the feeling of despair the patient induced in her, realized that this must be a communication the patient could not verbalize, and then gave words to it.

It has been said that projection represents a higher form of defense than projective identification when we come to consider personality development, and perhaps this is true in that it may represent a greater degree of individuation. But projection occurs at the cost of repression, and consequently of insufficient integration of certain disavowed aspects of the person's makeup. Projective identification may be a more primitive form of defense, or a more primitive mechanism, but certainly when it is dominant the aspect of object relatedness is better preserved. Now a small child has no words with which to communicate. He can communicate only by inducing a certain affective response in the other. If this affect is picked up by the mother and understood by her, she can give words to what she thinks the child is experiencing. This is also what we do as analysts when we try to understand what it is the patient is feeling. This is identification in another sense, the identification of a feeling state and giving words to it, naming it. If this is done it will help, I think, to maintain cohesiveness of structure rather than fragmentation, during the period that the child or the patient is learning to renounce certain gratifications. If the mother is someone who does not accept many aspects of herself, who has to project, who does not accept her greed, her ambivalence, her hate, or some other aspect of herself, she is not going to react empathically to the messages from the child, and the child is going to feel misunderstood and lonely. If this happens a great deal, it may lead to psychotic development.

Anne-Marie Sandler (Israel/U.K.).   I have been increasingly unhappy about the fact that although we discuss very important mechanisms we do not ask ourselves why they occur. We should remember that the motivation which makes us use those mechanisms stems from conflicts and from the avoidance of too much conflict. When we experience too great a level of conflict we feel anxious, guilty, confused, and have many other feelings as well. These feelings are unpleasant, and then we start using all the mechanisms we have been talking about. What worries me increasingly is that we seem to be trying to explain all these mechanisms by talking about what is good and what is bad and how, as Otto Kernberg has said, what is good is kept in and what is bad is put out, and so on. But what is eminently psychoanalytic is that we are always dealing with conflict and the painful feelings which arise from that conflict. So I liked it when Dr. Meissner said that if someone has completely accepted a passive role, but in her fantasy she is an aggressor, we then have a conflict. We have constantly to remind ourselves as psychoanalysts that we are treating our patients and verbalizing what happens on the basis of the idea of conflict and of the tendency not to want to bear conflict because it is unpleasant. We try to avoid pain, and that is why we use all the mechanisms that are being described.

Joseph Sandler.   I should like to add a personal note before we go on, and to state my disagreement with some of my colleagues. I think that everything which is said about projective identification being an early process runs the risk of being pure mythology. Perhaps things of that sort do go on very early in life, but we cannot really know whether or not the infant confuses himself with his objects. We can speculate about what goes on, but to equate the idea of early projective identification with the defense in which the boundaries between self and object play an extremely important part, and in which the identification that occurs is an unconscious identification, is to my mind a mistake. Consciously what is felt in projective identification is that something is "not me," and to equate that process of putting something over the boundary with the hypothetical, almost magical early process called projective identification does not really explain to us how boundaries are formed. It sounds very nice to say that one projects, and then one takes something back, and then projects again, and that makes for boundaries. Perhaps it is like that, but to equate the earlier processes with the later ones is a mistake, and I believe that the distinction between the two ought to be maintained.

Otto Kernberg.   I'll start out with the last comment, and although I haven't consulted with Betty Joseph, she might agree on this one with me. First of all, I am very much in agreement with Anne-Marie Sandler when she says that when we talk about intrapsychic life of the sort that is relevant for our psychoanalytic work we always talk about conflict. I am totally in agreement with that, and to see the child as the passive victim of what happens to it is to ignore completely the complex intrapsychic reactions of the child to whatever or whoever might be victimizing him. The problem arises, I think, that in traditional ego psychology, particularly in the United States, conflict was seen as something occurring between the ego, the superego, and the id. It was seen as intersystemic, and the idea had not been fully developed that conflicts could be seen as intrasystemic, within the ego-id matrix, as conflicts that predate the differentiation into the tripartite structure of the mind. There are many people who will talk about prestructural conflict as being conflict between inside and outside, between child and environment, and I think that this is a gross mistake. From that point of view I am very much in agreement with Anne-Marie Sandler.

Turning now to Joseph Sandler, he states that we cannot talk about projective identification very early.

Joseph Sandler.   We *can* talk about it, but I do not think it is the same thing as the later use of projective identification as a defense.

Otto Kernberg.   It seems to me that you are touching on the question of whether there is differentiation between self and nonself from the beginning of life or not. I imagine that Betty Joseph thinks that there is such a differentiation from the beginning of life, and that there is activation of what she might call libido and aggression shown as "good" and "bad" affect states among other things, and that these enter immediately into conflict. So from her viewpoint I would assume that she would see no reason why introjection and projection in a weak sense, or projective identification in a strong sense, should not be operating from birth on.

If, on the other hand, one assumes, as I do, that there is a symbiotic state at the beginning, that at the beginning of life there is not yet a differentiation between self and nonself, we can raise the question of whether there can be projective identification at such a stage. I would say that there cannot be, but I would suggest that the origin of projective identification may be the effort to expel into the periphery an intolerable "bad state" as part of an effort to recover a good state of feeling, one which must exist at least in a fleeting memory. That could be seen as the prototype of conflict, the attempt to recover a good state and to escape from a bad one. It is not yet intrapsychic in that there is not yet a differentiation between inside and outside, but it is what we might call the template out of which intrapsychic conflict develops. I would, of course, agree that this is all theoretical speculation, and I could without difficulty produce five reasons why Betty Joseph is right and I am wrong, but I will not do this. I would rather let her do it.

I want to respond to one of Dr. Chayes's points about projection and projective identification. I think projection, as I see it, is a mechanism that develops later, and that projective identification is more primitive. This is a view that I have suggested in a number of publications, and would like to spell it out more clearly in the context of this discussion. Projection in the weak sense is, of course, there from very early on, as part of the process of trying to distinguish our inside from the outside: I have no problem with that, but projection in its common sense of attributing to someone else something that one cannot recognize any more in oneself is an advanced neurotic mechanism that requires repression. It is highly sophisticated and comes after projective identification, which is the more primitive mechanism predominating in psychotic and borderline patients. I think I am on solid clinical ground here. But all this doesn't mean that projective identification cannot be seen in people like those sitting at this table. It occurs during adolescence because of the development of identity crises at that age. We can also see it at points of severe regression in analysis, even with normal and neurotic people, in people who have a neurotic personality organization. Finally, it is particularly evident in the naive participant in unstructured group situations that undercut some of the ordinary intrapsychic supports of ego identity. Such group situations uncover the underlying disposition towards identity diffusion that remains as the counterpart of primitive object relations and defensive mechanisms, and it is therefore in those group situations where all of us tend to activate projective identification, among other mechanisms.

Rivka Eifermann (Israel). I feel I have learned a lot from people's clinical examples about the way they use projective identification in relation to transference. I also enjoyed the clinical examples very much from another point of view, in that they brought to life the enormous advances we have made in the use of ourselves in our work with patients. We could see again and again what tremendous steps we have made from the days of Freud, who thought that as analysts we should be a mirror to our patients and that countertransference was something we should get rid of. But at the same time, because the clinical illustrations were so impressive, I became concerned that perhaps they cover up some other aspect of our work. I should like to illustrate this very briefly with a small example from one of the patients Betty Joseph presented. She described T, the teacher, as saying "he spoke of me as a very fine analyst and I was flattered in such ways." He tried to flatter the analyst, but then immediately and repeatedly felt invaded. He felt that he took over the analyst's capacities. He distorted what the analyst said, and what he felt about it was that she being old, "felt threatened by this intelligent young person." Now it was very clear that Betty Joseph did not feel threatened at all. When she described how he thought he could change his profession and become an analyst, Betty Joseph responded to that idea. She smiled when she was talking about it. She also said, in a similar vein, that this patient does not inspire much envy. I think that she was unconsciously responding to his feeling of being threatening to her. This is a very small example, and it is not important whether I am accurate about it or not. The point I want to make is that we are all human. We have our fights in politics and within our Societies. Much of the time we are not conscious of our responses to others, but what has been completely ignored in this conference, precisely because there is so much emphasis on our improving our sensitivity to patients, is that much of the time we are not sensitive to our responses. We each carry our unconscious into the consulting room just as we carry it around with us all the time, and much of what goes on between us and the patient, and a great deal of our response of our patients, remains unconscious and will forever remain so. We all accept the idea that even if we are analyzed very thoroughly we still remain with our own unconsciouses, and I think that this is something which should be emphasized because it has implications for what we consider within the analytic situation and for what we do with our patients. What is the meaning, in the context of the analytic situation, of reaching the truth? There is a dialogue between two people, and this dialogue evolves over some years into a common memory—the patient influences my memory and I influence his. We evolve a common language that is ours, and a rather private narrative develops and redevelops between us. What we reconstruct might be of great help to the patient, but it is not necessarily historical truth that we reach together. These points about our limits as analysts have recently been emphasized by Schafer and Spence, and have not been brought up at all in this conference.

Leslie Sohn (U.K.).   The emphasis in the presentations and in our discussion has been about putting something into somebody else. As I remember the original thoughts on projective identification in the British Society, they contained a particular facet of thinking, namely that projective identification was seen as a defense against intolerable envy and as an outcome of a hatred of dependence. A part of the ego would split off and take over a particular function or capacity of a particular object or part object. So the end result of such a procedure would be, "I have what he, she, or it has, or I have some capacity of that particular object." The end result is that one is identified either with the object or with the capacity of the object. I think that clarifies why the term identification enters into projective identification. The nature of the identification is, of course, highly precarious.

Having listened to the discussion, particularly to the contributions of Otto Kernberg, I should like to take him up on the question of "into" or "onto." I cannot believe that Otto Kernberg projected his epistemophilic impulses *onto* the wide theory that he has so beautifully presented to us. He must have projected them *into* the theory, right inside it, because we have shared with him the results of these projections of his creative mind. So please, Dr. Kernberg, try "into." This may open further areas of the mind, particularly in the clinical area. We have all kept very quiet in this colloquium about our technical differences. Each of the members of the panel would have produced very different reports of the first case Otto Kernberg presented. There are technical differences in regard to waiting, timing, rethinking, and restructuring, and I am pretty certain that if Betty Joseph would have presented one of the other analyst's patients, the interventions would have occurred much earlier. The question of where and when the interpretations begin reflects our clinical differences, and until we can have a profound examination of the differences in technique between us, I don't think we will get anywhere.

Joseph Sandler.   I am inclined to agree with Dr. Sohn in that the theories on which we really base our clinical practice are formed in parallel with what we do, and even as a consequence of what we do, and we may not be aware of these theories. What we present publicly is to a very large degree rationalization, identification with group standards, and so on. It would certainly be very worth our while to look at the differences between us in regard to what we actually do in the clinical situation.

Eva Basch-Kahre (Sweden). We have had a lot of theorizing, and some people say they know what projective identification is, while others say that it doesn't really exist. So I think we should first find out how it exists for different people. I have personally experienced projective identification many times in my consulting room, although it could easily have been called something else. The simplest form is when a patient says that he feels the analyst is angry with him today, but actually the patient is angry himself. And then there is the patient who projects his feelings into the analyst, and that is when one suddenly feels very sad, aggressive, or angry regarding the patient without finding any reason for it. The most primitive kind of projective identification I have experienced is when I have suddenly felt very tired, almost going to sleep, a state of mind that I believe is caused when the patient is projecting something very primitive into the analyst, something Bion would call beta elements. I am not sure that I am right, but I am giving these experiences in order to provide something concrete.

Joseph Sandler. Of course there isn't such a *thing* as projective identification, but there are certain phenomena which are not adequately encompassed by the other concepts we have and use. What has developed within psychoanalytic thinking has been a broad notion of projective identification that does seem to fit these additional phenomena, in many different ways. Clearly the term is used to refer to a very early process in the infant in which the process helps to establish boundaries between self and nonself, and to deal with intolerable affects. Obviously if there were no intolerable feelings the infant wouldn't develop at all. The concept has also been used for the process of making the analyst sad or angry, and I would say that the analyst who gets tired, to use the example quoted a little earlier, may get tired because the patient has pushed some tiredness into him. He may also, of course, be tired because he didn't get much sleep the night before, or because the patient is actually very boring. You could say that the patient is being aggressive with his boringness, and in that way what happens is projective identification. Well, that may be true sometimes. Projective identification is also used for the externalization of a superego introject, which isn't the same as the projection of an aspect of the self-representation. It is used to encompass all sorts of manipulation of other people. Now to say that this is simply projection onto the analyst as a mirror, a distortion of the image of the analyst, is not enough. Quite clearly patients induce feelings, thoughts, and attitudes in the analyst. This is done in various ways, and I tend to think in terms of manipulation, of what I have called "role responsiveness," and so on, but I am quite happy nowadays to have this brought under the umbrella notion of projective identification. But I want to stress that projective identification is not one thing.

Shirley Love (U.S.A.).   The concept of projective identification is a useful and sound one, and in connection with it I want to discuss the idea of the paranoid-schizoid position. I am interested in the process of interpretation to patients who are fixated at this very early and primitive level of development. Betty Joseph has referred to the limitations of interpretation with such patients, and I wonder whether there are communications other than interpretations, which are not threatening to the ego, and which can be more easily digested and absorbed than verbal communications.

Sidney Love (U.S.A.).   I want to give an example which I think may bear on the question of projective identification. An eleven-year-old girl asks, in her interview, whether I am more interested in her or in the money her family pays me. I asked her about her feelings, but she said she would not tell me because it would hurt me too much. Now the problem in that family was that the parents were making millions of dollars, and valued making money more than caring for their children. The child could not express her hurt feelings about this situation, so she put the whole family situation into the question she asked me. She identified with the hurting parents and made me the hurt child. Later she could verbalize more clearly the hurt she felt in regard to her mother and father for neglecting her. From a technical point of view, I think it more appropriate to start by asking patients what they are feeling when they ask the sort of question this eleven-year-old asked than to interpret to them, to tell this girl, for instance, that she feels hurt by her parents.

Rafael Moses.   The mechanisms we have been talking about go into operation in response to a conflict, and it is extremely important for us to remember this. We would probably all agree on that point. From a technical point of view, we would also probably agree that we would focus or zero in on an affective communication above everything else. I agree with Joseph Sandler's formulation about the way patients induce things in us, and I think it is true that patients prompt us, in one way or another, to assume one particular role or another. But as an analyst I cannot say that when I work with my patients I can locate projective identification all the time. I don't think we can assume that there is always projective identification going on, and that it is only a question of our allowing ourselves to become aware of it and to respond to it. Here there are technical differences between different schools, and at times this leads people to believe that what *they* do is better than what others do. In regard to the question of things going on in us that we remain forever unaware of, I am reminded of one of the examples I gave. We can have different people taking on the function of the two opposing sides in a conflict; or the two members of a couple might have an unconscious, implicit agreement that they take on the different sides of a conflict, and they may stick to this. This is something that happens very often, and may continue until some forceful change occurs. What I want to refer to is what occurs when one of the partners is lost, or changes his or her point of view, and this forces the other to become more aware of the two sides of the conflict, and therefore to take more responsibility for the conflict. Now we might hope that people can arrive at this by working on themselves, but I don't think that we can expect this to happen in ordinary life. But in an analytic situation I would want to see such processes occurring much more.

Betty Joseph. When Mrs. Love and Dr. Sidney Love spoke of making communications to one's patient that are not threatening, then I think of what has been a very important shift in our technical approach. We have become more sensitive to the existence of transference and countertransference, of the feelings that are occurring in both patient and analyst, and we try more to notice which part of the patient's personality we can most constructively talk to. So rather than just trying to analyze what has been said by these very disturbed patients, we try to interpret to the patient in such a way as to talk to that part that is able to listen to us, that can see what he is doing.

I think I can see what Dr. Basch-Kahre means when she says that she discovers in her work that she can explain certain things only by assuming the existence of projective identification. Many of us feel that.

I thought that Rivka Eifermann's contribution was very sensitive. She is right when she speaks of feeling that all the while so much goes on between patient and analyst that we can never take it for granted that we know everything that is going on. However, we must always try to see what is happening, and of course we should also listen to what the patient is actually saying. There is a danger that the importance we have placed on projective identification might easily lead us to underestimate the importance of the actual verbal communication of the patient.

To come back to the big issue of the distinction between projective identification and projection, and the whole connection of these with conflict, I found myself completely in agreement with Anne-Marie

Sandler. It seems to me to be most important to look at our understanding of projection and projective identification in relation to the conflict with which, from my point of view, the child is born. The child has to adjust to an outside world and to adjust to impulses that are in conflict. Now if we want to talk generally in terms of a child or infant projecting, we are making use of an umbrella term. But from the beginning the child doesn't just project into a vacuum but projects into an object. Naturally, those who feel that the child is not in a relationship with an object at the beginning would not agree with me, and there must be an essential difference of opinion about this in a group as large as this. Such differences are immaterial as long as we do not gloss them over. From my point of view the child projects *into* an object, and I would call this projective identification, seeing it as occurring from the beginning of life. I cannot understand how the child would get a feeling about the nature of its mother unless its own feelings were going into the mother and toward the mother. This must, to my mind, color the picture of the mother. It would take a much more grown-up child to be able to tell what the mother was *really* like.

Joseph Sandler. I once heard Herbert Rosenfeld say at the British Society that when the child cries it is putting its distress into the mother, and that that was projective identification. I must say my mind boggled when I heard him say that. What I do know is that the child cries because it is in distress, and I think we have to take certain biological "givens" into account. The mother reacts, contains the distress if you will, deals with the child, and out of that a world of interaction is built. This is a different way of looking at things, but unfortunately we don't have time to go into that today.

Otto Kernberg. I want to express my agreement with what Dr. Sandler has just said. As I see it, Betty Joseph is right in that the child relates to the mother from the beginning of life; but, as Winnicott pointed out, one has to differentiate the objectivity of that relationship from the subjective structures which are developing in the infant, and which require particular developmental preconditions. But we all agree here that there are different developmental models, and that it would be very interesting to discuss them further.

My conclusion is that we are in agreement as to the definition of projective identification, at least clinically, in that it is a dominant mechanism that can be seen particularly in patients who are rather ill. Such patients are those with borderline personalities and psychotic personality organizations. Even if we do not accept that the mechanism may be widespread, it is particularly clear and significant in patients like these, and it includes all the components we have identified. From this viewpoint projective identification is a very important, specialized type of projection, the definition and clinical use of which represents significant progress in our understanding of the transference and how to handle it. It seems to me that we also agree, from a technical point of view, on the importance of openness to our countertransference. In this regard I think it is good news that there is at least one area in which we have come to agree, namely, the definition of countertransference and its clinical use. Twenty years ago there were bitter fights around the traditional concept that countertransference should be defined as the unconscious reaction of the analyst to the transference of the patient, but now we see countertransference reactions as part of a broader concept that also includes realistic reactions to the transference and to other aspects of the patient's life as well as the analyst's. Countertransference is a broad spectrum of reactions. Within that spectrum, what is induced by the patient as part of projective identification is important. The analyst has to protect his internal freedom for exploring countertransference reactions within himself, for fantasying about the patient, and then must use his countertransference in formulating his interpretations. What he should *not* do is simply to communicate his countertransference to the patient. All of this represents an important technical development over the past twenty years.

My final point is that while clinically we can afford to let our concepts be loose and flexible, from the point of view of the development of psychoanalysis it is important that we try to make our concepts more precise.

W. W. Meissner. Well, in conclusion, I want to make two brief points that may be overlapping or interconnected. The first is that I have come to this seat of ancient wisdom in the person of a man from Missouri. We have a saying in the United States that when somebody says "I'm from Missouri" that means, "Man, you got to show me. I ain't gonna believe nothing if I don't see the facts." Well, the man from Missouri here has to say that in reviewing the case material he has heard, he ain't seen it yet. Neither Betty Joseph's cases, which were splendid clinical examples, nor in those of Otto Kernberg, whose luminosity is no less, have I found material that speaks to me of projection identification. What I read and hear are projections followed by introjections, and when I ask myself if anything more is being said, I am not satisfied with the answers I hear. Now the closest thing that I heard to projective identification came from Dr. Sohn, who described what he thought it was, who told us what the projection was and what it was about and what the identification was. Now *that* I can hear very clearly, and if he wishes to call it projective identification I have no problem with it. What he doesn't tell us is whether in fact what he is referring to is a process in which some part of the self is placed in that other object, and then identified with, or whether he is in fact entertaining a fantasy of having a capacity that, let us say, another object possesses. Similarly, when Dr. Kernberg says to Dr. Sandler, "You think like I do," what is happening? Is it projection? Is it projective identification? Or has Dr. Kernberg simply misunderstood Dr. Sandler? Obviously it is a form of primitive mirroring that is taking place, but we really don't know what the mechanism is. So we need to get at the facts.

The second point I want to make is that what we have been listening to for several days is what, with all due respect to my esteemed colleagues, I would call psycho-babble. Now I choose the word advisedly because it is psychoanalytic talk, but for all practical purposes it is babble. It is infantile talk. We are very much in a situation in psychoanalysis where our concepts lack sophistication. We are struggling with very complex phenomena with a very limited vocabulary with which to express and interpret our experiences. Now perhaps Dr. Kernberg will in future years lead us in this crusade, and we may be able to achieve greater definition and delineation in our concepts, greater exactitude in our language, but as yet we are stuck with primitive words. So when Dr. Kernberg says "projection" I am not at all sure what he means until he points it out in the clinical material. Then I can say, "Oh, that's what he's talking about." Or if Betty Joseph labels something projective identification I don't know what she means. I have to wait until she actually tells me what happened in the concrete situation. Then I can make some connection with it. I hope that with time and genius we may be led to richer fields, but in the meantime I think we are stuck with psycho-babble.

Joseph Sandler.   Just a few words of babble. Perhaps we *are* in a tower of Babel. We are certainly all tired, and quite clearly our honeymoon about projective identification came to an end just before our proceedings did. But I hope that some degree of cross-fertilization will have taken place without too much artificial insemination. It remains for me only to thank the participants in this conference wholeheartedly—both speakers and audience—for their participation in what was at the very least a most rewarding experience.

References

Abraham, K. (1924), A short study of the development of the libido viewed in the light of mental disorders. In: *Selected Papers on Psycho-Analysis*. London: Hogarth Press. 1927, pp. 418–501.

Ackerman, N. W. (1958), *The Psychodynamics of Family Life*. New York: Basic Books.

Allport, G. W. (1958), *The Nature of Prejudice*. New York: Doubleday.

Alphasi, I. (1974), *Hasidism* (Hebrew). Tel Aviv: Ma'ariv.

Ansky, S. (1926), *The Dybbuk*. New York: Boni & Liveright.

Appleman, S. (1979), *The Jewish Woman in Judaism*. Hicksville, NY: Exposition Press.

Ashkenazi, S. (1953), *The Woman in Jewish Tradition* (Hebrew). Tel Aviv: Izra'el.

Bellak, L. (1950), On the problem of the concept of projection. In: *Projective Psychology*, ed. L. E. Abt & L. Bellak. New York: Knopf.

Ben-Yehuda, N. (1980), The European witch craze of the 16th to 17th centuries: A sociological perspective. *Amer. J. Sociol.*, 86(11):1–31.

Biber, M. (1946), The maiden of Ludmir (Hebrew). *Rashumot*, 2:69–76.

Bick, E. (1968), The experience of the skin of early object-relations. *Internat. J. Psycho-Anal.*, 49:484–486.

Bilu, Y. (1979), Sigmund Freud and Rabbi Yehudah: On the Jewish mystical tradition of "psychoanalytic" dream interpretation. *Psychological Anthropol.*, 2(9):443–463.

––––––– (1980), The Moroccan demon in Israel: The case of "evil spirit disease." *Ethos*, 8(1):24–39.

––––––– (1985), The taming of the deviants and beyond: An analysis of "dybbuk" possession and exorcism in Judaism. *The Psychoanalytic Study of Society*, 11:1–31.

Bion, W. R. (1961), *Experiences in Groups*. London: Tavistock.

––––––– (1962), *Learning from Experience*. London: Heinemann.

––––––– (1963), *Elements of Psycho-Analysis*. London: Heinemann.

––––––– (1967), *Second Thoughts: Selected Papers on Psycho-Analysis*. London: Heinemann.

––––––– (1974), *Brazilian Lectures 1: Sao Paulo, 1973*, ed. J. Salomao. Rio de Janeiro: Imago Editora.

––––––– (1975), *Brazilian Lectures 2: Rio/Sao Paulo, 1974*, ed. J. Salomao. Rio de Janeiro: Imago Editora.

Bourguignon, E., Ed. (1973), *Religion, Altered States of Consciousness and Social Change*. Columbus: Ohio State University Press.

––––––– (1976), *Possession*. Corta Madera, CA: Chandler & Sharp.

––––––– (1981), Belief and experience in folk religion: Why do women join possession trance cults? Lecture presented at the Interdisciplinary Folklore/Religion Symposium: Faith and Belief, Ohio State University.

Brodey, W. W. (1965), On the dynamics of narcissism: I. Externalization and early ego development. *The Psychoanalytic Study of the Child*, 20:165–193. New York: International Universities Press.

197

Bychowski, G. (1956), The release of internal images. *Internat. J. Psycho-Anal.*, 37:331–338.

Crapanzano, V. (1977), Introduction. In: *Case Studies in Spirit Possession*, ed. V. Crapanzano & V. Garrison. New York: Wiley.

_____ Garrison V., Eds. (1977), *Case Studies in Spririt Possession*. New York: Wiley.

Eder, M. D. (1933), The Jewish phylacteries and other Jewish ritual observances. *Internat. J. Psycho-Anal.*, 14:341–375.

Edgcumbe, R. (1976), Some comments on the concept of the negative oedipal phase in girls. *The Psychoanalytic Study of the Child*, 31:35–61. New Haven, CT: Yale University Press.

Eidelberg, L. (1938), Pseudo-identification. *Internat. J. Psycho-Anal.*, 19:321–330.

Eissler, R. (1953), Scapegoats of society. In: *Searchlights on Delinquency*, ed. K. Eissler. New York: International Universities Press, pp. 288–305.

Emde, R. N., Kligman, D. H., Reich, J. H., & Wade, T. D. (1978), Emotional expression in infancy. In: *The Development of Affect*, ed. M. Lewis & L. Rosenblum. New York: Plenum.

Fairbairn, W. R. D. (1941), A revised psychopathology of the psychoses and psychoneuroses. *Internat. J. Psycho-Anal.*, 22:250–279.

Fenichel, O. (1925), Introjection and the castration complex. In: *The Collected Papers of Otto Fenichel: First Series*. New York: Norton, pp. 39–70.

_____ (1926), Identification. In: *The Collected Papers of Otto Fenichel: First Series*. New York: Norton, pp. 97–112.

_____ (1946), *The Psychoanalytic Theory of Neurosis*. London: Routledge & Kegan Paul.

Ferenczi, S. (1909), Introjection and transference. In: *Contributions to Psycho-Analysis*. Boston: Richard G. Badger, 1916.

_____ (1912), On the definition of introjection. In: *Final Contributions to the Problems and Methods of Psycho-Analysis*. London: Hogarth Press, 1955.

Fliess, R. (1953), Countertransference and counteridentification. *J. Amer. Psychoanal. Assn.*, 1:268–284.

Freud, A. (1936), *The Ego and the Mechanisms of Defense*. New York: International Universities Press.

_____ (1965), *Normality and Pathology in Childhood*. New York: International Universities Press.

Freud, S. (1887–1902), *The Origins of Psycho-Analysis*. New York: Basic Books, 1954.

_____ (1896), Further remarks on the neuro-psychoses of defence. *Standard Edition*, 3:162–185. London: Hogarth Press, 1962.

_____ (1900), The Interpretation of Dreams. *Standard Edition*, 4/5. London: Hogarth Press, 1953.

_____ (1905), Three essays on the theory of sexuality. *Standard Edition*, 7:130–253. London: Hogarth Press, 1953.

_____ (1911), Psycho-analytic notes upon an autobiographical account of a case of paranoia (dementia paranoides). *Standard Edition*, 12:9–79. London: Hogarth Press, 1958.

_____ (1912–1913), Totem and taboo. *Standard Edition*, 13:1–161. London: Hogarth Press, 1955.

_____ (1914), On narcissism: An introduction. *Standard Edition*, 14:73–102. London: Hogarth Press, 1957.

_____ (1915a), A case of paranoia running counter to the psycho-analytic theory of the disease. *Standard Edition*, 14:263–272. London: Hogarth Press, 1957.

_____ (1915b), Instincts and their vicissitudes. *Standard Edition*, 14:117–140. London: Hogarth Press, 1957.

_____ (1915c), The unconscious. *Standard Edition*, 14:166–215. London: Hogarth Press, 1957.

_____ (1916-1917), Introductory lectures on psycho-analysis. *Standard Edition*, 15/16. London: Hogarth Press, 1963.

_____ (1917), A metapsychological supplement to the theory of dreams. *Standard Edition*, 14:222–235. London: Hogarth Press, 1957.

_____ (1918), From the history of an infantile neurosis. *Standard Edition*, 17:7–122. London: Hogarth Press, 1955.

_____ (1920), Beyond the pleasure principle. *Standard Edition*, 18:7–64. London: Hogarth Press, 1955.

_____ (1921), Group psychology and the analysis of the ego. *Standard Edition*, 18:69–143. London: Hogarth Press, 1955.

_____ (1922), Some neurotic mechanisms in jealousy, paranoia and homosexuality. *Standard Edition*, 18:223–232. London: Hogarth Press, 1955.

_____ (1923), The ego and the id. *Standard Edition*, 19:12–66. London: Hogarth Press, 1961.

_____ (1924), The economic problem of masochism. *Standard Edition*, 19:159–170. London: Hogarth Press, 1961.

_____ (1926), Inhibitions, symptoms and anxiety. *Standard Edition*, 20:87–174. London: Hogarth Press, 1959.

_____ (1927), The future of an illusion. *Standard Edition*, 21:5–56. London: Hogarth Press, 1961.

_____ (1930), Civilization and its discontents. *Standard Edition*, 21:64–145. London: Hogarth Press, 1961.

_____ (1931), Female sexuality. *Standard Edition*, 21:225–243. London: Hogarth Press, 1961.

_____ (1933a), New introductory lectures on psycho-analysis. *Standard Edition*, 22:5–182. London: Hogarth Press, 1964.

_____ (1933b), Sandor Ferenczi. *Standard Edition*, 22:227–229. London: Hogarth Press, 1964.

_____ (1933c), Why war? *Standard Edition*, 22:203–215. London: Hogarth Press, 1964.

_____ (1937), Analysis terminable and interminable. *Standard Edition*, 23:216–253. London: Hogarth Press, 1964.

_____ (1939), Moses and monotheism. *Standard Edition*, 23:7–137. London: Hogarth Press, 1964.

_____ (1940), An outline of psycho-analysis. *Standard Edition*, 23:144–207. London: Hogarth Press, 1964.

_____ (1941), Findings, ideas, problems. *Standard Edition*, 23:299–300. London: Hogarth Press, 1964.

Fuchs, S. H. (1937), On introjection. *Internat. J. Psycho-Anal.*, 18:269–293.

Furman, E. (1980), Transference and externalization in latency. *The Psychoanalytic Study of the Child*, 35:267–284. New Haven, CT: Yale University Press.

Goodman, F. D. (1981), *The Exorcism of Anneliese Michel*. Garden City, NY: Doubleday.

Greenbaum, L. (1973), Societal correlates of possession trance in sub-Saharan Africa. In: *Religion, Altered States of Consciousness and Social Change*, ed. E. Bourguignon, Columbus: Ohio State University Press.

Greenson, R. R. (1954), The struggle against identification. *J. Amer. Psychoanal. Assn.*, 2:200–217.

Grinberg, L. (1957), 'Perturbaciones en la interpretación por la contraidentificación proyectivas. *Rev. de Psicoanál.*, 14.

—— (1958), 'Aspectos mágicos en la transferencia y en la contratransferencia: Identificación y contra identificación proyectivas. *Rev. de Psicoanál.*, 15.

—— (1962), On a specific aspect of countertransference due to the patient's projective identification. *Internat. J. Psycho-Anal.*, 43:436–440.

—— (1979), Projective counteridentification and countertransference. In: *Countertransference*, ed. L. Epstein & A. H. Feiner. New York: Aronson, pp. 169–191.

—— Sor, D., & de Bianchedi, E. T. (1977), *Introduction to the Work of Bion*. New York: Aronson.

Grossman, W. I. (1982), The self as fantasy: Fantasy as theory. *J. Amer. Psychoanal. Assn.*, 30:919–938.

Grotstein, J. (1982), *Splitting and Projective Identification*. New York: Aronson.

Guntrip, H. (1952), The schizoid personality and the external world. In: *Schizoid Phenomena, Object Relations and the Self*. London: Hogarth Press, 1968.

Haley, J., & Hoffman, L. (1967), *Techniques of Family Therapy*. New York: Basic Books.

Hartmann, H. (1939), *Ego Psychology and the Problem of Adaptation*. New York: International Universities Press.

Heimann, P. (1950), On counter-transference. *Internat. J. Psycho-Anal.*, 31:81–84.

—— (1952), Functions of introjection and projection. In: *Developments in Psycho-Analysis*, ed. M. Klein, P. Heimann, S. Isaacs, & J. Riviere. London: Hogarth Press, pp. 122–168.

Hendrick, I. (1936), Ego development and certain character problems. *Psychoanal. Quart.*, 5:320–346.

Hoffman, M. L. (1978), Toward a theory of empathic arousal and development. In: *The Development of Affect*, ed. M. Lewis & L. Rosenblum. New York: Plenum.

Horodetsky, S. A. (1944), *Hasidism and Its Teachings* (Hebrew). Tel Aviv: Dvir.

Horney, K. (1926), The flight from womanhood: The masculinity complex in women, as viewed by men and women. *Internat. J. Psycho-Anal.*, 7:324–339.

Isaacs, S. (1948), The nature and function of phantasy. *Internat. J. Psycho-Anal.*, 29:73–97.

Jacobson, E. (1957), Denial and repression. *J. Amer. Psychoanal. Assn.*, 5:61–92.

—— (1964), *The Self and the Object World*. New York: International Universities Press.

Jaffe, D. S. (1968), The mechanism of projection: Its dual role in object relations. *Internat. J. Psycho-Anal.*, 49:662–677.

Jaques, E. (1955), Social systems as a defence against persecutory and depressive anxiety. In: *New Directions in Psycho-Analysis*, ed. M. Klein, P. Heimann, & R. Money-Kyrle. London: Basic Books, pp. 478–498.

Kernberg, O. (1965), Notes on countertransference. *J. Amer. Psychoanal. Assn.*, 13:38–56.

—— (1975), *Borderline Conditions and Pathological Narcissism*. New York: Aronson.

—— (in press), The dynamic unconscious and the self. In: *Theories of the Unconscious*, ed. R. Stern. Hillsdale, NJ: Analytic Press.

Klein, M. (1929), Personification in the play of children. In: *Love, Guilt and Reparation and Other Works: 1921–1945*. London: Hogarth Press, 1975, pp. 248–257.

—— (1930), The importance of symbol-formation in the development of the ego. In: *Love, Guilt and Reparation and Other Works: 1921–1945*. London: Hogarth Press, 1975, pp. 219–232.

_____ (1931), A contribution to the theory of intellectual inhibition. In: *Love, Guilt and Reparation and Other Works: 1921-1945*. London: Hogarth Press, 1975, pp. 236-247.

_____ (1932), *The Psycho-Analysis of Children*. London: Hogarth Press.

_____ (1935), A contribution to the psychogenesis of manic-depressive states. In: *Love, Guilt, and Reparation and Other Works: 1921-1945*. London: Hogarth Press, 1975, pp. 262-289.

_____ (1946), Notes on some schizoid mechanisms. *Internat. J. Psycho-Anal.*, 27:99-110.

_____ (1952), The origins of transference. In: *Envy and Gratitude and Other Works: 1946-1963*. London: Hogarth Press, 1975, pp. 48-56.

_____ (1955), On identification. In: *Envy and Gratitude and Other Works: 1946-1963*. London: Hogarth Press, 1975, pp. 141-175.

_____ (1963), On the sense of loneliness. In: *Envy and Gratitude and Other Works: 1946-1963*. London: Hogarth Press, 1957, pp. 300-313.

_____ (1975a), *Envy and Gratitude and Other Works, 1946-1963*. London: Hogarth Press.

_____ (1975b), *Love, Guilt and Reparation and Other Works: 1921-1945*. London: Hogarth Press.

_____ Heima , P., & Money-Kyrle, R., Eds. (1955), *New Directions in Psycho-Analysis*. London: Tavistock.

Klepholtz, I. (1972), *The Admors of Belze* (Hebrew). Bnei-Brak: Pe'er HaSefer.

Knight, R. P. (1940), Introjection, projection and identification. *Psychoanal. Quart.*, 9:334-341.

Lacks, R. (1980), *Women and Judaism: Myth, History and Struggle*. Garden City, NY: Doubleday.

Laplanche, J., & Pontalis, J. B. (1973), *The Language of Psychoanalysis*, trans. D. Nicholson-Smith. London: Hogarth Press.

Le Bon, G. (1920), *The Crowd: A Study of the Popular Mind*. New York: Viking Press, 1960.

Lewis, I. M. (1966), Spirit possession and deprivation cults. *Man*, 1:307-329.

_____ (1971), *Ecstatic Religion: An Anthropological Study of Spirit Possession and Shamanism*. Baltimore: Penguin.

Lidz, T. (1965), *Schizophrenia and the Family*. New York: International Universities Press.

Loewald, H. W. (1961), Comments on some instinctual manifestations of superego formation. In: *Papers on Psychoanalysis*. New Haven, CT: Yale University Press, 1980.

_____ (1962), Internalization, separation, mourning, and the superego. In: *Papers on Psychoanalysis*. New Haven, CT: Yale University Press, 1980.

_____ (1980), *Papers on Psychoanalysis*. New Haven, CT: Yale University Press.

Lubin, A. J. (1958), A feminine Moses. *Internat. J. Psycho-Anal.*, 39:535-546.

Malin, A., & Grotstein, J. S. (1966), Projective identification in the therapeutic process. *Internat. J. Psycho-Anal.*, 47:26-31.

Meissner, W. W. (1970), Notes on identification: I. Origins in Freud. *Psychoanal. Quart.*, 39:563-589.

_____ (1978a), The conceptualization of marriage and family dynamics from a psychoanalytic perspective. In: *Marriage and Marital Therapy: Psychoanalytic, Behavioral and Systems Theory Perspectives*, ed. T. J. Paolin & B. S. McGrady. New York: Brunner/Mazel.

_____ (1978b), *The Paranoid Process*. New York: Aronson.

_____ (1980), A note on projective identification. *J. Amer. Psychoanal. Assn.*, 28:43-67.

————— (1981), *Internalization in Psychoanalysis*. New York: International Universities Press.

Mills, J. (1979), *Six Years with God*. New York: A & W.

Mintz, J. R. (1968), *Legends of Hasidism*. Chicago: University of Chicago Press.

Money-Kyrle, R. E. (1956), Normal countertransference and some of its deviations. *Internat. J. Psycho-Anal.*, 37:360–366.

Moses, R. (1978), Some psychic trauma: The question of early disposition and some detailed mechanisms. *Internat. J. Psycho-Anal.*, 59:353–364.

————— (1982), The group self and the Arab-Israeli conflict. *Internat. Rev. Psycho-Anal.*, 9:55–65.

————— (1983a), Emotional response to stress in Israel: A psychoanalytic perspective. In: *Stress in Israel*, ed. S. Bresnitz. New York: Van Nostrand Reinhold.

————— (1983b), Guilt feelings in political process. *Sigmund Freud Bulletin* (Vienna), 7(1):2–14.

————— (1984), Dehumanization of the victim and of the aggressor. Unpublished manuscript.

————— Halevi, H. (1972), A facet analysis of the defense mechanism of projection. Unpublished manuscript.

Nigal, G. (1983), *Dybbuk Stories in Jewish Literature* (Hebrew). Jerusalem: Rubin Mass.

Novick, J. & Kelly, K. (1970), Projection and externalization in latency. *The Psychoanalytic Study of the Child*, 25:69–95. New York: Quadrangle.

Nunberg, H. (1955), *Principles of Psychoanalysis*. New York: International Universities Press.

Obeyesekere, G. (1970), The idiom of demonic possession: A case study. *Social Study & Medicine*, 4:97–111.

Oesterreich, T. K. (1930), *Possession, Demoniacal and Other*. New York: Richard R. Smith.

Ogden, T. H. (1979), On projective identification. *Internat. J. Psycho-Anal.*, 60:357–373.

————— (1982), *Projective Identification and Psychotherapeutic Technique*. New York: Aronson.

Ornston, D. (1978), On projection: A study of Freud's usage. *The Psychoanalytic Study of the Child*, 33:117–166. New Haven, CT: Yale University Press.

Patai, R. (1978), Exorcism and xenoglossia among the Safed Kabbalists. *J. Amer. Folklore*, 91:823–835.

Racker, H. (1953), A contribution to the problem of countertransference. *Internat. J. Psycho-Anal.*, 34:313–324.

————— (1957), The meaning and uses of countertransference. *Psychoanal. Quart.*, 26:303–357.

————— (1968), *Transference and Countertransference*. New York: International Universities Press.

Rangell, L. (1980), *The Mind of Watergate*. New York: Norton.

Rapaport, D. (1952), Projective techniques and the theory of thinking. In: *The Collected Papers of David Rapaport*, ed. M. M. Gill. New York: Basic Books, 1967, pp. 461–469.

————— (1967), A theoretical analysis of the superego concept. In: *The Collected Papers of David Rapaport*, ed. M. M. Gill. New York: Basic Books.

Redl, F. (1966), *When We Deal With Children*. Glencoe, IL: Free Press.

Rosenfeld, H. (1952), Notes on the superego conflict in an acute schizophrenic patient. *Internat. J. Psycho-Anal.*, 33:111–131.

———— (1964), On the psychopathology of narcissism: A clinical approach. *Internat. J. Psycho-Anal.*, 45:332–337.

———— (1965), *Psychotic States: A Psycho-Analytical Approach.* New York: International Universities Press.

———— (1971), A clinical approach to the psychoanalytic theory of the life and death instincts: An investigation into the aggressive aspects of narcissism. *Internat. J. Psycho-Anal.*, 52:169–178.

———— (1975), Negative therapeutic reaction. In: *Tactics and Techniques in Psychoanalytic Therapy: Vol. 2. Countertransference*, ed. P. L. Giovacchini, New York: Aronson.

———— (1978), Notes on the psychopathology and psychoanalytic treatment of some borderline patients. *Internat. J. Psycho-Anal.*, 59:215–221.

———— (1983), Primitive object relations and mechanisms. *Internat. J. Psycho-Anal.*, 64:261–267.

Sadan, D. (1938), *From the Region of Childhood* (Hebrew). Tel Aviv: Davar.

Sandler, J. (1960), On the concept of superego. *The Psychoanalytic Study of the Child*, 15:128–162. New York: International Universities Press.

———— (1961), Identification in children, parents and doctors. In: *Psychosomatic Aspects of Paediatrics*, ed. R. MacKeith & J. Sandler. London: Pergamon.

———— (1976a), Actualization and object relationships. *J. Phila. Assn. Psychoanal.*, 3(3):59–70.

———— (1976b), Countertransference and role-responsiveness. *Internat. Rev. Psycho-Anal.*, 3:43–47.

———— (1983), Reflections on some relations between psychoanalytic concepts and psychoanalytic practice. *Internat. J. Psycho-Anal.*, 64:35–45.

———— (1985), *The Analysis of Defense: The Ego and the Mechanisms of Defense Revisited* (with A. Freud). New York: International Universities Press.

———— (1986), Comments on the self and its objects. In: *The Emergence and Development of Self and Object Constancy*, ed. S. Bach, J. A. Burland, & R. Lax. London: Guilford Press, pp. 97–106.

———— Dare, C. (1970), The psychoanalytic concept of orality. *J. Psychosom. Res.*, 14:211–222.

———— Joffe, W. G. (1967), The tendency to persistence in psychological function and development, with special reference to fixation and regression. *Bull. Menn. Clin.*, 31:257–271.

———— Kennedy, H., & Tyson, R. L. (1975), Discussions on transference: The treatment situation and technique in child psychoanalysis. *The Psychoanalytic Study of the Child*, 30:409–441. New Haven, CT: Yale University Press.

———— ———— ———— (1980), *The Technique of Child Analysis.* London: Hogarth Press.

———— Rosenblatt, B. (1962), The concept of the representational world. *The Psychoanalytic Study of the Child*, 17:128–162. New York: International Universities Press.

———— Sandler, A. -M. (1978), On the development of object relationships and affects. *Internat. J. Psycho-Anal.*, 59:285–296.

———— ———— (1984), The past unconscious, the present unconscious and interpretation of the transference. *Psychoanalytic Inquiry*, 4:367–399.

Schafer, R. (1968), *Aspects of Internalization.* New York: International Universities Press.

———— (1972), Internalization: Process or fantasy? *The Psychoanalytic Study of the Child*,

27:411–436. New York: Quandrangle.

Scheidlinger, S. (1952), *Psychoanalysis and Group Behavior*. New York: Norton.

Scholem, G. (1971), Gilgul. In: *Encyclopedia Judaica*, 7:573–577. Jerusalem: Keter.

Searles, H. (1951), Data concerning certain manifestations of incorporation. In: *Collected Papers on Schizophrenia and Related Subjects*. New York: International Universities Press, 1965, pp. 39–69.

———— (1965), *Collected Papers on Schizophrenia and Related Subjects*. New York: International Universities Press.

Segal, H. (1973), *Introduction to the Work of Melanie Klein*. London: Hogarth.

Shapiro, D. S. (1965), *Neurotic Styles*. New York: Basic Books.

Singer, I. B. (1959), *Satan in Gorey*. New York: Noonday Press.

Stern, D. N. (1983), Affect attunement. In: *Frontiers of Infant Psychiatry*, ed. J. D. Call, E. Galenson, & R. L. Tyson. New York: Basic Books, 1984.

Strachey, A. (1941), A note on the use of the word "internal." *Internat. J. Psycho-Anal.*, 22:37–43.

Thorner, H. (1955), Three defences against inner persecution. In: *New Directions in Psychoanalysis*, ed. M. Klein, P. Heimann, & R. Money-Kyrle. London: Tavistock, pp. 282–306.

Tversky, Y. (1949), *The Maiden of Ludmir* (Hebrew). Jerusalem: Mosad Bialik.

Volkan, V. (1979), *War and Adaptation: A Psychoanalytic History of Two Ethnic Groups in Conflict*. Charlottesville, VA: University of Virginia Press.

Vogel, E. F., & Bell, N. W. (1960), The emotionally disturbed child as the family scapegoat. In: *The Family*, ed. N. W. Bell & E. F. Vogel. Glencoe, IL: Free Press.

Waelder, R. (1951), On the structure of paranoid ideas. *Internat. J. Psycho-Anal.*, 32:167–177.

Walker, S. S. (1972), *Ceremonial Spirit Possession in Africa and Afro-America*. Leiden: E. G. Brill.

Weiss, E. (1939), The psychic presence. *Bull. Menn. Clin.*, 3:177–193.

———— (1947), Projection, extrajection and objectivation. *Psychoanal. Quart.*, 16:357–377.

———— (1960), *The Structure and Dynamics of the Human Mind*. New York: Grune & Stratton.

Winnicott, D. W. (1958), *Collected Papers*. London: Tavistock.

Wynne, L. (1965), Some indications and contraindications for exploratory family therapy. In: *Intensive Family Therapy*, ed. I. Boszormenyi-Nagy & J. L. Framo. New York: Harper & Row.

Zborowski, M., & Herzog, E. (1962), *Life Is with People: The Life of the Shtetl*. New York: Schocken.

Zinner, J. (1976), The implications of projective identification for marital interaction. In: *Contemporary Marriage: Structure, Dynamics and Therapy*, ed. H. Grunebaum & J. Christ. Boston: Little, Brown.

———— Shapiro, R. (1972), Projective identification as a mode of perception and behaviour in families of adolescents. *Internat. J. Psycho-Anal.*, 53:523–530.

Name Index

Subject Index

Printed in the United States
by Baker & Taylor Publisher Services